KT-172-143

COMMON MEDICAL EMERGENCIES

A GUIDE FOR JUNIOR PHYSICIANS

COMMON MEDICAL EMERGENCIES

A GUIDE FOR JUNIOR PHYSICIANS

By

R. H. SALTER, B.Sc., M.B., B.S.(Lond.), M.R.C.P.

Senior Medical Registrar, Bristol Royal Infirmary

REPRINT

BRISTOL

JOHN WRIGHT & SONS LTD

1968

© JOHN WRIGHT & SONS LTD., 1968

Distribution by Sole Agents:
United States of America: The Williams & Wilkins Company, Baltimore
Canada: The Macmillan Company of Canada Ltd., Toronto

First edition September, 1968
Reprinted August, 1969
Reprinted October, 1970

ISBN O 7236 209 03

PRINTED IN GREAT BRITAIN BY JOHN WRIGHT AND SONS LTD.,
AT THE STONEBRIDGE PRESS, BRISTOL

PREFACE

FROM the patient's point of view, admission to hospital for any reason is usually a frightening experience. Emergency admission is particularly alarming and the patient requires continual reassurance and calm, confident handling by the receiving hospital doctor.

However, the latter is usually a house-officer serving his pre-registration year who may be seeing many of the medical emergencies, with which he is expected to deal competently, for the first time.

Supervision by more senior medical staff is often not available when it is most needed and the experience may be almost as worrying for the house-officer as it is alarming for the patient.

The aim of the author, who is still closely concerned with the management of acute medical problems, has been to provide a book specifically to help junior house-physicians in the management of common medical emergencies, most of which are the cause of patients' admission to hospital, although some may occur during their stay as in-patients.

It is not intended to be comprehensive and the selection of conditions for consideration was based on an analysis of the causes of emergency admission to a general medical unit for acute cases over a 12-month period, those included comprising 95 per cent of all the conditions encountered.

Only emergency management has been considered, more experienced advice usually being available by the time decisions concerning maintenance therapy need to be taken.

References have not been quoted in the text but some suggestions for further reading have been included.

Bristol,   R. H. SALTER
    August, 1968.

CONTENTS

COMMON MEDICAL EMERGENCIES

A GUIDE FOR JUNIOR PHYSICIANS

Chapter I

MYOCARDIAL INFARCTION

MYOCARDIAL infarction presents few problems in diagnosis when the presentation is classical, i.e., the sudden onset of severe retrosternal chest pain, often described as a feeling of pressure or heaviness, radiating into the neck, jaws, back, or down the arms. Frequent additional features are sweating, nausea, vomiting, and a feeling of faintness. The pain is persistent and the patient usually obtains no relief until opiates are administered.

If left ventricular failure occurs the pain may occasionally be masked by the presence of severe breathlessness, the cause of the pulmonary oedema only becoming apparent after electrocardiography and serum enzyme determinations.

In the elderly, myocardial infarction may be painless, the patient complaining of nothing other than transient faintness or loss of consciousness, and unless further investigations are undertaken the potential seriousness of these apparently minor complaints will be missed.

Physical examination frequently reveals no abnormality but it is well worth listening carefully for the presence of pericardial friction and a third heart sound. Repeated auscultation is essential, for both these valuable signs may be short-lasting. Although occasionally low, the blood-pressure, contrary to popular belief, is usually normal and may even be elevated in the early stages of the illness.

As a result of the lack of physical signs, the diagnosis is usually made from the history, and the presence of retrosternal chest pain in a patient middle-aged or older should be treated with great caution. If such patients present at the Casualty Department it is far safer to admit them to hospital for observation and further investigation, than to discharge them merely because there are no abnormal physical findings and a single electrocardiogram reveals no pathological features.

The main differential diagnoses are causes of chest pain from thoracic structures other than the myocardium (pericardium, oesophagus, lungs and pleura, chest wall, aorta, nerve-roots) and the possibility of an intra-abdominal catastrophe. Although this is a lengthy list, diagnosis is rarely difficult after careful history-taking and a thorough physical examination.

Confirmatory Evidence

The electrocardiogram (E.C.G.) is by far the most valuable investigation, for the result is available immediately. The main features of a transmural myocardial infarction are deep Q waves, elevation of the S-T segment in leads facing the damaged area with reciprocal S-T depression in remote leads and steep symmetrical T wave inversion. However, it must be realized that these changes may take up to several days to develop, and serial tracings are essential in cases of doubt. For this reason, as already stated, clinical impressions are of paramount importance and if, from the history alone, a patient is thought to have sustained a myocardial infarction he should be confined to bed despite an initial negative E.C.G. Subsequent daily tracings will be required and other confirmatory evidence sought, the latter consisting mainly of:—

1. A slight elevation of the temperature occurring 24–48 hours after admission and persisting for several days.

2. Haematological evidence of muscle necrosis, i.e., an elevated E.S.R. and a polymorph leucocytosis.

3. Serum enzyme determinations: these are not necessary if the E.C.G. is diagnostic, but if it is normal, the abnormalities only minor, or the tracing difficult to interpret because of a previous infarct, digitalis therapy, or the presence of left bundle-branch block, they may be of great value. Blood should be taken at the time of admission and again after 24 hours for the estimation of serum glutamic oxaloacetic transaminase (S.G.O.T.). This usually reaches its peak level 24 hours after a myocardial infarction but may remain elevated for at least 48 hours.

The advantage of the serum lactic dehydrogenase (S.L.D.H.) is that the maximum value of this enzyme does not usually occur until 48–72 hours after the infarct. Thus, if a patient has sustained an infarction one or two days before his admission to hospital, the peak level of the S.G.O.T. might be missed, whereas the S.L.D.H. would probably still be significantly elevated.

Unfortunately, neither the E.C.G. abnormalities nor the serum enzyme elevations described are absolutely specific for myocardial damage and it is worth stressing again that all these investigations might be negative and yet the patient have suffered a major myocardial infarction. This explains both why so much care is needed before dismissing the complaint of central chest pain in a person aged 40 or over as of no serious significance and the advisability of relying so heavily on clinical impressions.

MANAGEMENT

Pain relief is vital, and an opiate is usually required for this purpose. The use of morphine is traditional, and 10–15 mg. intramuscularly should be given on admission if the patient is still complaining of pain, or 5 mg. intravenously if severely distressed. Unfortunately, morphine is a potent emetic, and it is wise to give 50 mg. intramuscularly of either cyclizine or chlorpromazine routinely when prescribing this drug. Heroin is less likely to induce vomiting and is a more potent analgesic than morphine, 10 mg. being a suitable intramuscular dose. Injections of either drug should be repeated until the pain is relieved, and frequent large doses may be required. The possibility of addiction to these opiates following such short-term administration is extremely small and such a remote risk should not prohibit their prescription in adequate dosage. A serious side-effect of both morphine and heroin is respiratory depression, and for this reason these drugs should be used with caution for patients who, in addition, suffer from chronic obstructive airways disease.

The place of anticoagulants has not been finally decided. Although of doubtful effectiveness as far as the infarct itself is concerned, there is no doubt that the incidence of thrombo-embolic complications is reduced, and unless there are any obvious pre-existing sources of haemorrhage, patients in the younger age-group (up to 65 years) with myocardial infarction should be given anticoagulant treatment irrespective of the severity of the attack. Intravenous heparin is given after the diagnosis has been confirmed, 40,000 units being added to a litre of 5 per cent dextrose in distilled water and infused over 24 hours. At the same time 40 mg. of warfarin are given orally followed by 5 mg. after 48 hours. The heparin infusion (40,000 units daily) can be discontinued after 48 hours and the subsequent dose of warfarin controlled by estimation of the prothrombin time.

COMPLICATIONS

The main complications of myocardial infarction associated with an increase in mortality are:—

1. Arrhythmias and conduction disorders (see Table I).
2. Hypotension.
3. Cardiac failure.
4. Thrombo-embolism.

1. ARRHYTHMIAS AND CONDUCTION DISORDERS

Although a shrewd guess as to the nature of an arrhythmia can often be made by examining the arterial pulse, careful inspection of the jugular venous pulsation, auscultation, and the effects of carotid compression, an E.C.G. is essential for accurate diagnosis. Ideally, continuous E.C.G. monitoring should be available for the first 72 hours after admission, to enable any potentially serious arrhythmias which occur to be detected and corrected at the earliest opportunity. For this reason it is desirable that all patients with myocardial infarction should be admitted initially to a coronary care unit; there is no doubt that the introduction of these units has lowered the mortality from this condition. As yet, however, such units are few, and the most that can be offered in their absence is careful ward observation and the correction of any factors which might facilitate the occurrence of an arrhythmia, e.g., anoxia, digitalis overdosage.

Sinus tachycardia reflects the severity of the infarction or its complications, and there is no specific treatment.

Digoxin, 0·5 mg. initially, followed by 0·25 mg. at 6-hourly intervals, is indicated both for rapid persistent atrial fibrillation and also for persistent atrial tachycardia when there is no possibility of digitalis overdosage.

Frequent ventricular ectopics predispose to ventricular tachycardia and fibrillation, and for that reason should be treated with either oral procainamide 250 mg. 6-hourly or oral propranolol in doses of up to 30 mg. every 4 hours.

Table I.—ARRHYTHMIAS AND CONDUCTION DISORDERS AFTER MYOCARDIAL INFARCTION

	ARTERIAL PULSE	MAIN E.C.G. FEATURES	MANAGEMENT
Sinus tachycardia	Rapid Regular	Normal complexes Rapid rate	No specific treatment
Atrial fibrillation	Rapid Irregular	Irregular but normal QRS complexes. P waves replaced by fibrillation waves	Digoxin if arrhythmia persistent
Atrial tachycardia	Rapid Regular	Rapid normal QRS complexes preceded by abnormal P waves	Digoxin if arrhythmia persistent (and not precipitated by digitalis overdosage)
Ventricular ectopics	Basically regular with frequent premature beats	Basically sinus rhythm but frequent bizarre QRS complexes with no preceding P waves	Oral procainamide or propranolol
Ventricular tachycardia	Rapid Regular	Rapid regular QRS complexes of bizarre form resembling the appearances in bundle-branch block	Intravenous lignocaine, procainamide, or propranolol. Electrical conversion if sinus rhythm not quickly resumed
Ventricular fibrillation	Absent	Irregular, bizarre, or atypical complexes	External cardiac massage and assisted ventilation. Electrical defibrillation
Complete heart block	Slow Regular	Regular P waves occurring independently of slow normal QRS complexes	Electrical pacing with an intracardiac electrode

Ventricular tachycardia is potentially lethal and requires urgent treatment with either intravenous lignocaine (up to 50 mg.), intravenous procainamide (up to 1·0 g.), or intravenous propranolol (up to 5 mg.). All these drugs should be injected extremely slowly, under continuous E.C.G. control, and with careful observation of the blood-pressure. Electrical conversion with a synchronous d.c. defibrillator is easy and safe, and its use should not be delayed if reversion to sinus rhythm is not quickly obtained.

Cardiac arrest, due either to asystole or ventricular fibrillation, is treated initially by external cardiac massage and mouth-to-mouth respiration. After tracheal intubation, ventilation with pure oxygen is commenced. The nature of the arrhythmia is established by electrocardiography and correction attempted either by the use of a d.c. defibrillator or, in the case of asystole, by pacing with an intracardiac electrode. The metabolic acidosis, which rapidly occurs as the result of tissue under-perfusion, is corrected with adequate amounts of intravenous bicarbonate, 100 mEq. being a suitable initial dose.

The occurrence of complete heart-block with myocardial infarction is associated with a particularly high mortality. If the slow ventricular rate results in hypotension, heart failure, or Stokes-Adams attacks, pacing with an intracardiac electrode is indicated, but facilities for this procedure are not generally available. Unfortunately, drug therapy is not particularly effective but isoprenaline in the highest tolerated doses 4-hourly together with a diuretic and corticosteroids should be tried.

2. HYPOTENSION

Persistent hypotension after myocardial infarction is usually indicative of a poor prognosis, and the mortality remains high, despite all forms of treatment. For cardiogenic shock vasoconstrictor drugs are contra-indicated and intravenous hydrocortisone is usually ineffective. Oxygen at high concentration should be given, metabolic acidosis due to tissue hypoxia corrected by intravenous infusion of bicarbonate, and any arrhythmia corrected if possible.

3. CARDIAC FAILURE

Mild left ventricular failure is a frequent occurrence after myocardial infarction and, even though the clinical evidence may be minimal, results in a significant reduction of arterial oxygen tension by impairing oxygen up-take in the lungs. Thus, oxygen therapy and a diuretic are indicated if this complication is suspected. The recognition and management of severe pulmonary oedema is outlined in the following chapter.

4. THROMBO-EMBOLISM

Thrombosis of a deep leg vein is a recognized complication of myocardial infarction, and thrombus may also form on the endocardium overlying the necrotic heart muscle. Embolism may occur from either of these sites, a factor which constitutes the main justification for the use of anticoagulants in this condition. Deep vein thrombosis is discussed more fully in Chapter IV and some of the consequences of embolism in Chapters III, V, and XI.

Summary

1. The diagnosis of myocardial infarction is based primarily on the history, with particular reference to the nature, site, intensity, and radiation of the chest pain. However, painless infarction may occur (particularly in the elderly), or the pain be obscured by the manifestations of acute left ventricular failure.

2. Physical signs are relatively uncommon. Transient pericardial friction or a gallop rhythm provide valuable supporting evidence when they occur.

3. The E.C.G. is usually abnormal but several days may elapse before the abnormality becomes manifest.

4. Estimation of S.G.O.T. and S.L.D.H. activity is particularly helpful when the E.C.G. abnormalities are minor or difficult to interpret.

5. Effective pain relief is essential, heroin being the drug of choice.

6. If admission to a coronary care unit is impossible, careful ward observation is vital.

7. Complications should be promptly dealt with as outlined.

Chapter II

ACUTE LEFT HEART FAILURE

WHEN the function of the right heart chambers remains unimpaired, failure of the left heart, either because of atrial or ventricular inadequacy, results initially in pulmonary venous congestion with an increase in pulmonary venous pressure. The increased hydrostatic pressure is transmitted to the pulmonary capillaries and pulmonary oedema occurs when the rapid transudation of fluid from the capillaries into the alveoli exceeds the reabsorptive capacity of the lymphatics. The pulmonary venous engorgement and presence of oedema fluid, both in the alveoli and connective tissue planes, result in a decrease of lung compliance, with the consequence that breathing requires an increased mechanical effort and the ventilation/perfusion relationships throughout the lung are disturbed. These abnormalities of respiratory function probably account for the dyspnoea which is the outstanding manifestation of left heart failure.

CAUSES OF LEFT HEART FAILURE

The common causes of left ventricular failure (*Fig.* 1) are :—

1. Systemic hypertension.
2. Ischaemic heart disease.
3. Aortic valve disease.
4. Mitral regurgitation.

Left atrial failure usually results from mitral stenosis.

Often a precipitating factor, such as anaemia, a lower respiratory tract infection, or the sudden development of an arrhythmia is responsible for the production of sudden left heart failure when the function of the chambers has already been seriously impaired by the basic disease process.

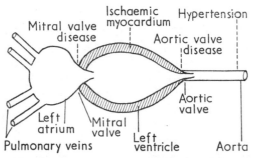

FIG. 1.—Common causes of acute left heart failure.

CLINICAL PICTURE

Dyspnoea is the outstanding symptom of left heart failure, occurring initially only on exertion but later also at rest and on lying flat.

Characteristically attacks of breathlessness occur during the night, the patient wakening with acute dyspnoea, often accompanied by a dry cough and a sensation of tightness across the chest. Severe retrosternal pain may be present if a myocardial infarction has occurred. Sitting up usually makes the breathing a little easier but frequently the patient rises from bed and walks to an open window to try and overcome the frightening sensation of suffocation. When pulmonary oedema occurs the dyspnoea is extremely severe and associated with the coughing of large amounts of thin, frothy, blood-stained sputum.

Physical examination reveals the patient to be extremely distressed, dyspnoeic, ashen, and cyanosed, with a cold clammy skin.

The three important signs of left heart failure are:—

1. *Fine crepitations* which may be generalized but are usually heard only at the lung bases. These occur only in the presence of pulmonary oedema and there may be no physical signs of pulmonary venous hypertension alone.

2. *Triple rhythm*, the additional heart-sound being proto-diastolic and indicative of a left ventricle under strain. A pre-systolic sound, resulting from left atrial hypertrophy, may also be audible. If the heart-rate is rapid it may be difficult to decide the origin of the additional sound, particularly as both sounds may be summated because of a shortened diastole. Auscultation is often difficult, due to the presence of sounds of respiratory origin, and triple rhythm is often easier to feel than hear.

3. *Pulsus alternans*, the rhythm being regular but with alternate strong and weak beats. This sign is often difficult to elicit by palpation but can easily be detected with a sphygmomanometer. As the cuff pressure is lowered, and at the point marking the systolic blood-pressure, only half the beats are audible over the brachial artery. When the pressure is lowered further, the remaining beats become audible so that the original pulse-rate is doubled.

The jugular venous pressure may or may not be elevated.

Signs of the underlying cardiovascular lesion will also be apparent.

DIFFERENTIAL DIAGNOSIS

Other important causes of acute dyspnoea from which left heart failure must be distinguished are:—

1. Acute laryngeal obstruction.
2. Sudden loss of functioning lung tissue, e.g., infarction, massive collapse, pneumothorax.
3. Reversible airways obstruction (bronchial asthma).
4. Severe haemorrhage.
5. Hysterical over-ventilation.

In practice the only one of these conditions which is liable to cause any confusion is bronchial asthma. An expiratory wheeze is the hall-mark of airway obstruction but wheezing may also be a feature of left heart failure if the bronchial lumen is reduced by mucosal oedema.

Helpful points in the differential diagnosis of bronchial asthma and left heart failure are:—

1. Asthmatic patients usually have a long history of similar episodes and expectorate tenacious mucoid or purulent sputum during or after the paroxysm. A first episode of dyspnoea in a middle-aged or elderly patient is likely to be cardiac in origin.

2. The wheeze in bronchial asthma is predominantly expiratory and auscultation of the lung fields reveals diffuse expiratory rhonchi. Fine basal crepitations are not usually heard as a result of pure airways obstruction but are frequently audible in the presence of left heart

failure. As a consequence of oedema of the bronchial mucosa, rhonchi may also be heard in the latter condition but are not usually confined to expiration.

3. The presence of pulsus alternans and triple rhythm suggests the dyspnoea to be of cardiac origin and this is supported by detecting signs of an underlying cardiovascular lesion.

These points are summarized in *Table II* (p. 47).

INVESTIGATIONS

When dealing with a severely distressed, dyspnoeic patient, symptomatic relief is urgent and to delay this while undertaking further investigations is heartless and usually unnecessary.

A chest radiograph during an acute attack of pulmonary oedema reveals fan-shaped mottling radiating out from the hila and either generalized cardiomegaly or isolated enlargement of either the left atrium or ventricle. However, this is not required to establish the diagnosis.

Electrocardiography should be performed after the breathlessness has been relieved and serial tracings may be required if there is any suspicion of a myocardial infarction.

More detailed investigation as to the cause of the acute pulmonary congestion can be postponed until after the emergency has been dealt with.

MANAGEMENT

The patient should be propped up in bed and given oxygen to breathe in high concentration. This can most easily be achieved with a face mask (e.g., the M.C. Mask) and an oxygen flow of 6–8 litres/minute.

Morphine is the drug of choice, 10–15 mg. being given intramuscularly or 5–10 mg. intravenously, together with 50 mg. intramuscularly of either cyclizine or chlorpromazine as an anti-emetic. Patients with acute left heart failure are often denied this drug by junior medical staff who, being unsure of their diagnosis and aware of the risk of giving morphine in severe bronchial asthma, prefer to rely on the effect of 0·25–0·5 g. aminophylline by slow intravenous injection. Although this usually produces some improvement in either condition it does not have such a dramatic effect as morphine in relieving the alarming dyspnoea produced by acute pulmonary congestion and oedema. Careful physical examination should enable the diagnosis of acute left heart failure to be made with comparative confidence, after which morphine can be administered without hesitation. The major contra-indication to this recommendation is the coexistence of chronic obstructive airways disease when the administration of morphine may precipitate respiratory failure. In this eventuality nalorphine is a specific morphine antagonist, a suitable initial dose being 5–10 mg. intravenously.

Diuretics are extremely helpful and the rapidly acting preparations which can be given intravenously, such as frusemide 20 mg., ethacrynic acid 50 mg., or chlorothiazide 0·5 g., are indicated. The two most potent and rapidly acting preparations, frusemide and ethacrynic acid, should not be administered too frequently to elderly patients for the profound diuresis and electrolyte loss which they induce may precipitate urea retention and serious depletion of both body sodium and potassium.

Digitalization is indicated but rarely urgent unless an extremely rapid supraventricular arrhythmia is responsible for the production of acute left heart failure. In the latter event digoxin should be given intramuscularly rather than intravenously, for it is difficult to be certain that the patient has not previously received digitalis in some form and if diuretics have recently been administered the possibility of hypokalaemia also exists. Usually the oral route is sufficient, a suitable régime being an initial dose of 1·0 mg. digoxin followed by 6-hourly doses of 0·25 mg. until the ventricular rate falls to below 100/minute.

Venesection is rarely necessary except in the condition of circulatory overload (*see below*).

Complete rest is essential; digoxin and a diuretic together with a potassium supplement should be continued in maintenance dosage. Morphine, 10–15 mg. subcutaneously, is often a useful hypnotic for the first night or two after admission to hospital because of acute pulmonary congestion.

Often neglected, although as important as the relief of the acute dyspnoea, is the subsequent treatment of the underlying cardiovascular lesion whenever this is possible.

CIRCULATORY OVERLOAD

This problem is encountered most frequently in medical wards and results from the occasional necessity of giving a blood transfusion to a patient with severe chronic anaemia. In these circumstances the blood-volume is normal, the cardiac output often considerably increased, and cardiac failure usually incipient. Blood transfusion may easily precipitate pulmonary oedema, particularly if the early indications of circulatory over-load (elevated jugular venous pressure, dry cough, dyspnoea, and a feeling of tightness across the chest), are ignored.

If acute pulmonary oedema does occur, treatment is as outlined, although venesection or the temporary trapping of blood in the legs by the use of sphygmomanometer cuffs applied to the thighs and inflated to mid-way between the systolic and diastolic pressure, may also be necessary.

This emergency can usually be prevented by:—

1. Using only packed cells instead of whole blood when transfusing chronically anaemic patients.

2. Transfusing only small volumes at a time and running the drip as slowly as possible.

3. Giving a potent diuretic, e.g., parenteral frusemide or ethacrynic acid, at the time of the transfusion.

4. Considering a form of exchange transfusion, where the patient's blood is removed from another vein in an equal amount to the volume of packed cells being transfused, if the precipitation of pulmonary oedema seems particularly likely.

SUMMARY

1. Although breathlessness with wheezing may be a feature of both acute left heart failure and bronchial asthma, these two conditions are rarely confused if:—

a. Attention is paid to the age of the patient and to the existence of previous similar episodes.

b. A careful examination is made for the three important signs of acute left heart failure, i.e., basal crepitations, triple rhythm, and pulsus alternans.

c. There is evidence of an underlying cardiovascular lesion.

2. Emergency management consists of:—

a. Sitting the patient up.

b. Oxygen in high concentration.

c. Morphine (unless there is associated chronic respiratory disease).

d. A rapidly-acting diuretic.

e. Intravenous aminophylline.

f. Digitilization.

3. The *cause* of the acute left heart failure should be treated whenever possible.

4. Pulmonary oedema from circulatory overload by over transfusing patients with chronic anaemia can largely be avoided by:—

a. Using only packed red cells.

b. Running the drip as slowly as possible.

c. Associated diuretic therapy.

Chapter III

ACUTE LOWER LIMB ISCHAEMIA

THE management of sudden occlusion of a major artery to the lower limb is essentially a surgical problem. Nevertheless, patients with this condition are frequently admitted to medical wards with the result that the responsibility for initiating treatment falls on the house-physician, although a surgical opinion should be obtained as soon as possible.

CAUSES OF ACUTE LOWER LIMB ISCHAEMIA

The commonest causes of sudden arterial occlusion in the leg are:—

1. The deposition of thrombus in a segment of an artery, the lumen of which is already narrowed by atheromatous intimal degeneration.

2. Embolism, usually from a thrombus in the left atrium in patients with mitral stenosis and atrial fibrillation, or from the left ventricle after a recent myocardial infarction, the thrombus having formed on the endocardium overlying the necrotic muscle. Occasionally fragments of thrombus and degenerate intima, which become detached from an atheromatous plaque higher up the arterial tree, may act as emboli and result in acute arterial occlusion more distally.

CLINICAL FEATURES

The patient invariably complains of the sudden onset of severe pain in the limb followed by a feeling of coldness and loss of power and sensation. Initially the leg appears white but unless a collateral circulation quickly develops this is replaced by cyanosis and mottling. The arterial pulses are absent beyond the site of occlusion.

DIAGNOSIS

The clinical features of acute lower limb ischaemia are so characteristic that the chances of its confusion with other causes of sudden severe leg pain are remote.

The decision as to whether the arterial occlusion is thrombotic or embolic in origin is more difficult. Embolism usually occurs with dramatic suddenness, a source for the embolus is evident, and a past history of circulatory impairment in the legs is unusual. Although thrombosis may also cause acute ischaemia there is usually a long history of intermittent claudication and physical examination reveals no source for an embolus.

The site of occlusion is usually easy to detect by palpation of the peripheral arteries and emergency arteriography is rarely necessary for this purpose.

MANAGEMENT

The treatment of sudden arterial occlusion of the lower limb is urgent, for if the blockage is not relieved gangrene will develop if the collateral circulation is inadequate.

Pain relief, for which frequent and large doses of morphine or pethidine are usually required, is essential and rapid heparinization (by the intravenous injection of 10,000 units followed by a continuous intravenous heparin infusion—40,000 units in 1 litre of 5 per cent dextrose over 24 hours) is indicated.

The ischaemic leg should be exposed and kept as cool as possible, to reduce the rate of metabolism of the tissues to a minimum, while the remainder of the body is

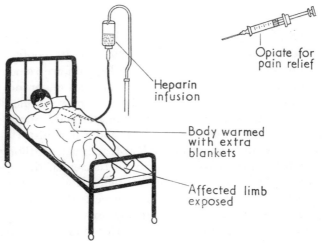

FIG. 2.—Management of acute lower limb ischaemia.

warmed to achieve maximal cutaneous vasodilatation, thus increasing blood-flow to the affected limb via the superficial vessels (*Fig.* 2).

Vasodilator drugs are of no value in these circumstances.

Thrombolytic therapy, using fibrinolytic agents by the intravenous or intra-arterial route, requires careful monitoring; its effectiveness has yet to be convincingly demonstrated.

A slow intravenous infusion of low molecular weight dextran (1 litre over 24 hours) may aid the circulation through the smaller vessels.

As already stated, however, surgery is the treatment of choice, particularly if an embolism is the cause of the occlusion. If both legs are involved and neither femoral pulse palpable (thus suggesting that the occlusion is at or near the aortic bifurcation), surgery should not be delayed.

If the occlusion is situated in a femoral artery, treatment is commenced as outlined above and the condition of the limb observed carefully for the next two hours. If the circulation does not show quick improvement, indicated by a pink flush, venous filling, and a gradual return of power and sensation, an operation to restore the circulation should be performed. A discussion of arterial surgery is beyond the scope of this book but it is important to note that modern techniques have made this a much less hazardous procedure than formerly and that the recent administration of heparin is no contra-indication to early operation. In consequence a patient should not be deprived of the chance of surgery because of coexisting cardiorespiratory disease without carefully considering the risks of continued conservative management. Similarly, the existence of the occlusion for several hours prior to the arrival of the patient at hospital is not an absolute contra-indication to operation, for successful restoration of function can be obtained after periods of ischaemia as long as 48 hours.

Summary

1. The characteristic clinical features of acute lower limb ischaemia are:—

   a. Sudden pain.

   b. Loss of sensation.

   c. Loss of power.

   d. Limb white initially, later mottled and cyanosed.

   e. Absent arterial pulses beyond the site of occlusion.

2. The distinction between an embolus and thrombosis can usually be made by the presence or absence of:—

   a. A source for an embolus.

   b. Previous circulatory impairment.

3. Emergency management consists of:—

   a. Pain relief.

   b. Immediate heparinization.

   c. Exposing the affected limb and warming the remainder of the body.

4. Arterial surgery should be considered if the circulation does not quickly improve within two hours of admission.

Chapter IV

DEEP VEIN THROMBOSIS

DEEP vein thrombosis is encountered most frequently in the lower limbs, the calf veins being the commonest site of origin, but thrombosis may also occur in the external iliac, common femoral, and profunda femoris veins.

The importance of this condition stems not from the local effect, although considerable morbidity may result from deep leg vein thrombosis (particularly if recurrent), but because of the possibility of thrombi becoming detached from their site of origin and transported in the blood-stream to the lungs with resulting pulmonary arterial obstruction (*see* Chapter V). Since pulmonary embolism may be fatal, thrombosis of a deep leg vein demands prompt and careful treatment.

The factors responsible for intravascular thrombosis are :—

1. An abnormality of the vein wall.
2. Diminished rate of blood-flow.
3. Increased coagulability of the blood.

These three causes were described by Virchow over 100 years ago and their importance has not yet been convincingly challenged.

Conditions with which an increased incidence of deep vein thrombosis is associated, and where the above factors operate either singly or in combination, are varicose veins, pressure from a pelvic tumour or gravid uterus, bed-rest, trauma, after surgery, cardiac failure, dehydration, polycythaemia, carcinoma (especially of the stomach, bronchus, and pancreas), and Buerger's disease. Nevertheless, in many cases there is no apparent predisposing cause.

Deep vein thrombosis of the lower limb is as likely to be encountered as a complication occurring in hospital in-patients as a cause for emergency hospital admission, and continued efforts both to prevent its occurrence and also for its early detection are essential if the incidence of pulmonary embolism is to be reduced.

CLINICAL FEATURES

Unfortunately thrombosis of a deep calf vein can occur without producing symptoms or signs, the first indication of its existence being the occurrence of a pulmonary embolus.

When symptoms do result from the thrombosis the patient usually complains of swelling and pain (which may amount to little more than a feeling of heaviness) in the affected leg.

Physical examination reveals the leg to be blue and swollen with pitting on pressure, the swelling being best confirmed by measurement of the calf or thigh. The skin is often shiny and warm and the superficial veins dilated. Calf tenderness is usually present and Homan's sign (pain in the calf when the calf muscles are stretched by dorsiflexion of the foot) may be positive. A higher venous occlusion is associated with more extensive swelling of the leg and tenderness can often be elicited over the course of the femoral vein.

If the patient is already in hospital, a small rise in the temperature and pulse-rate may be noted.

Diagnosis

When all the features described above are apparent the diagnosis presents no difficulty. However, the signs are often minimal and only enough to raise the suspicion of a deep vein thrombosis; in these circumstances it is usually safer to commence treatment rather than to do nothing and risk the subsequent occurrence of a pulmonary embolus. A deep vein thrombosis can be demonstrated by contrast radiography but this is rarely feasible as an emergency procedure.

There is little risk of its confusion with acute arterial occlusion for in deep vein thrombosis the leg is blue rather than white, and the arterial pulses are palpable, although occasionally reduced. A swollen leg after trauma may be due to bleeding into the soft tissues rather than to venous thrombosis and, if there is any doubt, an expert opinion should be obtained before anticoagulant therapy is commenced. Thrombophlebitis, in which the risk of pulmonary embolism is much less (although not completely absent), usually occurs in a superficial vein which is tender, often palpable as a subcutaneous cord, and there is overlying erythema.

The examination and investigation of the patient must also be directed to discovering a cause for the thrombosis; pelvic examination is particularly important if the femoral or iliac vein is involved.

MANAGEMENT

Treatment is primarily directed at preventing release and extension of the thrombus.

Unless there are any recognized contra-indications, anticoagulant therapy should be started immediately the diagnosis has been made. An intravenous infusion of heparin is commenced, (40,000 units in a litre of 5 per cent dextrose solution over a 24–hour period) and continued for 48 hours. Forty mg. warfarin are given on admission followed by 5 mg. after 48 hours. The subsequent daily dose of warfarin can then be regulated by serial estimations of the prothrombin time. Alternatively the heparin infusion may be continued for several days before it is replaced by warfarin, as there is good evidence that treatment with heparin is followed by a rapid improvement in the local clinical signs. However, prolonged heparin therapy should be monitored by frequent estimation of the clotting time and the dose adjusted so that this is maintained between 15 to 20 minutes.

The foot of the bed should be raised and the leg kept reasonably still except for gentle passive movements of the joints.

A mild analgesic, such as aspirin or paracetamol, is usually adequate for relief of the discomfort.

SUMMARY

1. Deep vein thrombosis is frequently not clinically apparent and a pulmonary embolus may be the first indication of its presence.

2. When clinically evident, one or more of the following physical signs may be present:—

a. Calf tenderness.

b. Positive Homan's sign.

c. Swelling of the leg with pitting oedema.

d. Skin blue and shiny.

e. Skin temperature increased.

f. Tenderness over the course of the femoral vein.

A high degree of suspicion is needed if the diagnosis is not to be missed.

3. Emergency management consists of:—

a. Heparinization.

b. Foot of bed elevated.

c. Relief of local discomfort.

Chapter V

PULMONARY EMBOLISM

THROMBI in the veins of the leg are by far the most important source of pulmonary emboli; hence the importance of the early recognition and treatment of deep vein thrombosis (*see* Chapter IV). It follows that pulmonary embolism occurs most frequently in patients who are particularly likely to develop leg vein thrombosis, e.g., after surgery, during pregnancy, in association with severe heart failure, prolonged bed-rest, etc. However, as stated in Chapter IV, extensive thrombosis of the leg veins may occur without any clinical evidence and also without any obvious precipitating factors. Youth is no protector and the occurrence of a massive pulmonary embolus in a young, apparently healthy, ambulant individual is well recognized.

The consequences of pulmonary embolism depend on many factors, e.g., the size of the embolus, whether previous pulmonary emboli have occurred, and the presence of coexisting cardiorespiratory disease. Death from massive pulmonary embolism is usually due to mechanical obstruction of the pulmonary circulation. Patients who survive the sudden impaction of a large embolus develop the features of circulatory obstruction. Smaller pulmonary emboli may cause only a transient fall in cardiac output or may be clinically silent and pass undiagnosed unless the signs and symptoms of pulmonary infarction become manifest later.

Pulmonary infarction is not an invariable consequence of embolism but is more likely to occur in the presence of pulmonary congestion, pleural effusion, pulmonary infection, and pulmonary collapse, and also if the emboli are multiple. Secondary infection, particularly with pneumococci, may result when the infarct is in a previously infected region of the lung.

CLINICAL FEATURES

These may best be considered under two headings:—
1. Massive pulmonary embolism.
2. Pulmonary infarction.

1. MASSSIVE PULMONARY EMBOLISM

Massive pulmonary embolism, if death is not immediate, results in acute shortness of breath with a sensation

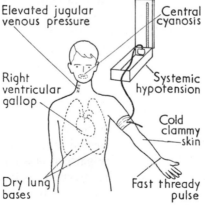

FIG. 3.—Signs of massive pulmonary embolism.

of tightness across the chest or severe retrosternal pain. Transient loss of consciousness or a feeling of faintness are common associated features. The sudden onset of these symptoms often occurs shortly after the patient has an urgent desire to defaecate.

The patient appears extremely agitated, breathless, and cyanosed, and the skin is cold and clammy. The arterial pulse is rapid and of poor volume and the blood-pressure usually falls. Signs of acute right heart strain may develop, i.e., an elevated jugular venous pressure and gallop rhythm, best heard in the 2nd or 3rd inter-space at the left sternal edge (*Fig.* 3).

2. PULMONARY INFARCTION

The characteristic features of pulmonary infarction are pleuritic pain and haemoptysis. When the infarct involves the diaphragmatic pleura the pain may be referred to the corresponding shoulder.

Chest examination is often unhelpful in the early stages although pleural friction or a few crepitations may be audible in the region of the infarct. A slight rise in temperature may occur in the first 24–48 hours and a pleural effusion is a frequent later development.

INVESTIGATIONS

1. PULMONARY EMBOLISM

In the absence of infarction, chest radiography is often unhelpful. Occasionally a clarified area in the lung field, due to a diminished vascular pattern and corresponding to the extent of the embolized artery, may be seen, or there may be evidence of cardiomegaly and dilatation of the main pulmonary artery. The diagnosis can be confirmed by pulmonary angiography but although this is a comparatively simple procedure it is not yet standard practice.

The E.C.G. is often normal but may reveal evidence of right axis deviation or right ventricular strain. A pattern similar to a posterior myocardial infarction may occur although a significant Q wave in Lead II rarely occurs in pulmonary embolism. However, the most useful E.C.G. feature which aids the differentiation between myocardial infarction and pulmonary embolism is that in the latter condition the abnormalities are transient, often lasting a few hours only, whereas the E.C.G. features of a myocardial infarction may last several weeks.

2. PULMONARY INFARCTION

Fever, a polymorph leucocytosis, and a raised erythrocyte sedimentation rate provide suggestive evidence of lung necrosis. An elevated serum L.D.H. level in the presence of normal S.G.O.T. activity favours pulmonary infarction but is not a specific feature of this condition.

A chest film may be normal in the early stages but frequently one or more of three radiological signs may be evident:—

a. An opacity produced by the infarction. Classically the shadow is triangular with the apex directed towards the hilum. Even when this is the case, however, the infarct may assume any shape when seen on a conventional postero-anterior film.

b. A small pleural effusion.

c. A raised diaphragm which moves poorly on respiration.

Diagnosis

The diagnosis of massive pulmonary embolism is comparatively easy in the presence of either clinical evidence of deep leg vein thrombosis or of predisposing factors to this condition. When neither of these are present, diagnosis is more difficult, since other cardio-vascular catastrophes may be closely simulated. The usual problem is to differentiate massive pulmonary embolism from myocardial infarction. Clinical features rarely aid their distinction other than a study of the jugular venous pressure. Although this may be elevated after a myocardial infarction, this is usually secondary to left heart failure and if the jugular venous pressure is raised in the presence of clear lung fields, pulmonary embolism is the most probable explanation.

As previously described, a chest radiograph and E.C.G. may be normal in the early stages and serial films and tracings are essential.

A dissecting aneurysm of the aorta can usually be excluded by clinical examination if the dissection involves the origin of the great vessels, and bacteraemic shock is distinguished by a low venous pressure, sur-prisingly warm, pink, peripheries, and a full-volume pulse, despite fairly severe systemic hypotension.

Respiratory emergencies, such as massive pulmonary collapse or a large pneumothorax, produce such gross and characteristic physical signs that their distinction from pulmonary embolism is no problem.

As for embolism, pulmonary infarction is easily diagnosed when pleuritic pain and haemoptysis occur in the presence of deep leg vein thrombosis or its predisposing factors. However, as extensive deep vein thrombosis may be clinically silent, the possibility of pulmonary infarction being the cause of any unexplained episode of pleuritic pain must be seriously considered. If untreated, further emboli may occur with the possibility of a fatal outcome. In practice, the main problem is to distinguish pulmonary infarction from infection. Pneumococcal pneumonia usually commences with a rigor and the sputum is rusty rather than blood-stained. Segmental collapse or less specific forms of pulmonary infection may cause confusion but the fact that the sputum is rarely purulent in the early stages of infarction is a helpful point. Unfortunately the radiographic features of pulmonary infarction are not specific and elevation of the serum L.D.H. in the presence of normal S.G.O.T. activity can certainly result from infection as well as infarction.

MANAGEMENT

1. MASSIVE PULMONARY EMBOLISM

Opiates are invaluable for the relief of pain, acute dyspnoea, and agitation. Either morphine 15 mg. intramuscularly (unless contra-indicated because of associated chronic respiratory disease) with parenteral cyclizine, or chlorpromazine as an anti-emetic, or pethidine 100 mg. intramuscularly are suitable.

Oxygen should be given in high concentration, this being obtained with a flow rate of 6–8 litres/minute and a suitable face mask, e.g., the M.C. mask.

Unless anticoagulants are contra-indicated a heparin infusion should be commenced, 40,000 units of heparin being added to 1 litre of 5 per cent dextrose solution and infused intravenously over 24 hours. Warfarin 40 mg. is given at the same time followed by 5 mg. after 48 hours. The heparin infusion can be discontinued after 36–48 hours and the subsequent dose of warfarin controlled by serial estimations of the prothrombin time.

Thrombolytic therapy with fibrinolytic agents needs careful monitoring and is not yet standard practice.

Vasoconstrictor drugs are not indicated for persistent systemic hypotension following massive pulmonary embolism. Unfortunately little can be done in these circumstances unless the circulatory obstruction is relieved. Since this necessitates embolectomy, this is often not feasible but the possibility of surgery should be considered if this complication occurs in a young, previously healthy person and if facilities for cardio-thoracic surgery are near at hand.

2. PULMONARY INFARCTION

Pethidine 50–100 mg. intramuscularly is usually necessary for pain relief and should be given without hesitation.

Unless contra-indicated, anticoagulant therapy should be commenced as outlined above, although the haemoptysis is likely to be intensified. Antibiotics may be given to prevent secondary infection of the infarct and oral administration is preferable to avoid the risk of haematoma formation from frequent intramuscular injections while receiving anticoagulants. Tetracycline, 250 mg. 6-hourly, or ampicillin 250–500 mg. 6-hourly, are both suitable for this purpose.

Occasionally a large pleural effusion is present at the time of admission and withdrawal of the fluid may be necessary.

SUMMARY

1. Pulmonary emboli almost invariably arise from thrombus in the deep veins of the leg or pelvis, whether or not this is clinically evident.

2. The initial manifestations of pulmonary embolism result from circulatory obstruction and, depending on the size and number of emboli, may vary from sudden death, acute breathlessness and cardiovascular collapse, to a syncopal attack. Small embolic episodes frequently pass unnoticed.

3. Pulmonary infarction, which is not an inevitable consequence of embolism, characteristically causes pleuritic pain and haemoptysis. Frequently however, haemoptysis does not occur and the pain is mild and short-lasting.

4. A chest radiograph, E.C.G., and estimation of S.L.D.H. activity are often informative but the diagnosis is not excluded if these investigations are negative.

5. The emergency management of massive pulmonary embolism consists of:—

   a. Oxygen in high concentration.
   b. Morphine.
   c. Heparinization.

6. The early treatment of pulmonary infarction consists of:—

   a. Pain relief (pethidine often necessary).
   b. Heparinization.
   c. Antibiotic to prevent secondary infection.

Chapter VI

SPONTANEOUS PNEUMOTHORAX

SPONTANEOUS pneumothorax is predominantly a disease of young, apparently healthy males, may be bilateral (although rarely simultaneously) and is often recurrent. There is usually no underlying lung pathology although spontaneous pneumothorax is also associated with chronic obstructive airways disease in later life.

The breach in the lung surface, probably due to the rupture of a small sub-pleural bleb or bulla, usually seals off rapidly, the air in the pleural cavity is absorbed, and the lung re-expands. Occasionally the defect remains open or may act as a one-way valve, allowing air to enter but not to escape from the pleural cavity with a consequent build-up of intrapleural pressure. This rare complication (tension pneumothorax) is potentially lethal for if the intrapleural pressure continues to increase, the mediastinum and great vessels may be so grossly displaced that asphyxia and circulatory collapse result.

CLINICAL FEATURES

The sudden onset of breathlessness and severe chest pain on the affected side are the characteristic symptoms, but if the air-leak is small the patient may be unaware of its occurrence. However, if ventilation is already seriously impaired from chronic obstructive airways disease, even a small pneumothorax may cause severe respiratory embarrassment.

Occasionally a loud extra clicking sound may be heard during the systolic phase of the cardiac cycle as a feature of a shallow left-sided pneumothorax. The click, which may be loud enough to be audible both to the patient and near-by observers, is probably due to the forcible separation of the visceral and parietal pleura during systole, when the air-pocket is in such a position that it can be moved by the cardiac pulsation.

If the pneumothorax is small, physical examination may be negative. Larger air-leaks may result in the chest wall on the affected side both moving less and appearing pushed forward, displacement of the mediastinum away from the affected side, hyperresonance on percussion, and diminished or absent breath sounds.

A tension pneumothorax results in extreme respiratory distress, gross mediastinal displacement, tachycardia, and a falling blood-pressure. Urgent treatment is required in these circumstances.

DIAGNOSIS

The diagnosis presents no problem when the air-leak has been large, for the clinical features are characteristic. Nevertheless the presence of a pneumothorax should be confirmed by a chest radiograph. This investigation is essential when the symptoms are suggestive but physical signs are lacking, and also when there is coexistent bronchial asthma or chronic obstructive airways disease. In the presence of these two conditions, even a small pneumothorax might precipitate severe breathlessness and is usually not detectable by clinical examination.

The characteristic appearance of a pneumothorax on a chest film is a thin line representing the lung edge, running internal to and parallel with the chest margin. Beyond this there is an area of increased translucency resulting from the absence of lung markings. When the pneumothorax is large the collapsed lung is seen compressed against the mediastinum which itself is displaced away from the affected side. A small pleural effusion is also frequently present.

In addition to the radiological features of the pneumothorax itself, the chest film will also reveal evidence of any underlying lung pathology although, as already stated, this is unusual.

MANAGEMENT

The pain from a spontaneous pneumothorax is often severe and pethidine 50–100 mg. intramuscularly is usually required for its relief. Oxygen is indicated if the patient is breathless and cyanosed, although the concentration may need to be carefully controlled if there is coexisting chronic obstructive airways disease (*see* Chapter VIII).

Whether it is necessary to remove the air from the pleural cavity depends on many factors. If the pneumothorax is of the tension type (indicated by extreme breathlessness, gross mediastinal displacement, and evidence of circulatory collapse) the air should be released immediately. A wide-bore needle inserted into the pleural cavity through the 2nd or 3rd interspace in the mid-clavicular line on the affected side will suffice in an emergency, although when the circumstances are less dramatic it is preferable to use an intrapleural catheter connected to an underwater seal.

In a previously healthy young adult, no intervention is needed if the lung is shown by the chest film to be less than 30 per cent collapsed. Careful observation is necessary and the initial decision may need reviewing if the lung does not quickly re-expand as expected. When the degree of pulmonary collapse is much greater, aspiration of the intrapleural air is advisable. The use of a soft rubber or latex catheter is preferable to a needle for the point of the latter may traumatize the lung surface when re-expansion occurs. Suitable sites for the introduction of an intra-pleural catheter are:—

1. The 2nd intercostal space in the mid-clavicular line. *Not Recom.*
2. The 4th intercostal space, high in the axilla.

Prior to the start of the manoeuvre it is wise to check that the catheter selected will run easily through the metal cannula. Then after the skin has been prepared, and under local anaesthesia, a small incision is made with a sharp-bladed scalpel through the skin and sub-cutaneous tissues. With a boring action the trocar and cannula are pushed through the chest wall. This is an unpleasant procedure for both the patient and operator as considerable pressure on the trocar is often required, particularly in young subjects with an elastic chest wall. When the chest wall is penetrated the trocar is withdrawn and a thumb quickly placed over the cannula. The catheter, with its distal end clamped by artery forceps, is then threaded through the cannula until a few centimetres are in the pleural cavity. The cannula is withdrawn enough to allow a further pair of artery forceps to be clamped across the catheter flush with the chest wall, the original pair of artery forceps removed and the cannula withdrawn completely. The catheter is then anchored firmly to the chest wall by strapping and connected to an underwater seal. The second pair of artery forceps is then removed, enabling air to escape from the pleural space without re-entering. Fluid, whether blood or a serous effusion, is also drained from the pleural cavity by this method.

In view of the remote risk of introducing infection into the pleural cavity by this procedure, a broad spectrum antibiotic, such as tetracycline 250 mg. 6-hourly, should be prescribed.

The criterion of the degree of pulmonary collapse is no guide to the necessity for active intervention in the presence of coexisting obstructive airways disease and conservative treatment is inappropriate in these circumstances even when the pneumothorax is small.

When the lung is collapsed passively, due to the presence of intrapleural air, sputum retention frequently occurs, with consequent atelectasis or absorption collapse. This complication should be prevented if possible by vigorous chest physiotherapy with as much postural coughing as the patient can tolerate.

SUMMARY

1. Spontaneous pneumothorax characteristically occurs in a young, apparently healthy male, causing acute breathlessness and chest pain.

2. Although clinical diagnosis is easy when the pneumothorax is large, physical examination may be negative if the air-leak is small and a chest radiograph is essential to establish the diagnosis.

3. There is usually no serious underlying lung lesion although there is an increased incidence of spontaneous pneumothorax in patients with acute or chronic obstructive airways disease.

4. Urgent reduction of intrapleural pressure is essential if the air in the pleural cavity is under tension.

5. Aspiration of the intrapleural air by an intercostal catheter is advisable if:—

a. The pneumothorax is large.

b. There is an associated haemothorax.

c. There is coexisting obstructive airways disease, in which case even a small pneumothorax can seriously impair ventilation.

Chapter VII

BRONCHIAL ASTHMA

BRONCHIAL asthma is defined clinically as paroxysmal shortness of breath associated with an expiratory wheeze. The mechanisms responsible for the variable airways obstruction (*see Fig. 4*), which is the cause of the breathlessness, are:—

1. Increased tone of the bronchial smooth muscle.

2. Thickening of the bronchial mucosa as a result of oedema or hyperaemia.

3. Plugging of the smaller airways by viscid secretions.

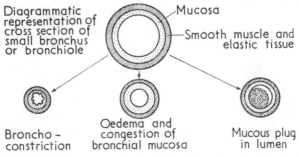

Fig. 4.—Mechanisms of variable airways obstruction. Diagrammatic representation of cross-section of small bronchus or bronchiole.

The major factors which precipitate asthmatic attacks are:—

1. Emotional disturbances.

2. Hypersensitivity.

3. Infection of the respiratory tract.

Patients with bronchial asthma are usually only admitted to hospital when the family doctor has been unable to relieve the condition in the home with conventional bronchodilator drugs, and the attack is thus usually already of several hours duration.

It was not formerly realized that hypoxaemia is a common occurrence even in mild asthmatic attacks. Severe bronchial asthma may cause dangerous hypoxaemia, hypercapnia, and acidosis, and is potentially lethal. In consequence, when the facilities are available, serial estimations of the arterial CO_2 and O_2 tensions should be performed if the patient's condition gives any cause for concern.

In the past, too much emphasis has been placed on bronchoconstriction as a cause of the generalized airways obstruction with consequent excessive reliance on so-called bronchodilator drugs for therapy. With the realization that the most striking pulmonary lesion in patients who die from this condition is widespread plugging of the bronchi and bronchioles with inspissated mucus, and the frequent clinical observation that asthmatic attacks terminate with the expectoration of sticky mucoid sputum, therapy has now been placed on a broader basis.

CLINICAL FEATURES

The predominant symptom is shortness of breath, associated with an expiratory wheeze. A viral upper respiratory tract infection is a common precipitating event, often resulting in a secondary bacterial bronchitis as indicated by a cough productive of purulent sputum. The patient usually complains of chest tightness but pain is not a feature.

There is usually a history of previous similar attacks, often dating back to childhood or early adult life.

Physical examination during a mild attack of bronchial asthma reveals a breathless patient with an audible expiratory wheeze, poor chest expansion, and diffuse expiratory rhonchi on chest auscultation. Other additional sounds are unusual although coarse crepitations may be audible in the presence of coexisting infection.

If the airways obstruction is severe the patient may be severely distressed, fatigued, pale, and cyanosed, with a fast pulse-rate and all accessory muscles of respiration in use.

If the condition is not relieved, respiratory and circulatory failure may develop. The danger signs, indicating that intensive therapy is urgent, are:—

1. Tachycardia.

2. The development of right heart strain as indicated by the development of gallop rhythm (heard at the lower left sternal edge in the third and fourth interspace) or E.C.G. features of acute cor pulmonale.

3. Minimum sputum production, suggesting the retention of secretions in the bronchial tree, further intensifying the airways obstruction.

4. Increasing restlessness and confusion, suggesting cerebral anoxia.

5. Increasing breathlessness with decreasing wheeze, indicating that the partial airways obstruction is becoming complete.

6. Exhaustion and evidence of peripheral circulatory failure.

DIAGNOSIS

The main condition likely to be confused with severe bronchial asthma is acute left heart failure, particularly as both frequently cause attacks of breathlessness during the night. Their differential diagnosis is considered in Chapter II and the helpful distinguishing points are listed in *Table II*.

Table II.—CLINICAL FEATURES AIDING DISTINCTION BETWEEN ACUTE LEFT HEART FAILURE AND BRONCHIAL ASTHMA

BRONCHIAL ASTHMA	ACUTE LEFT HEART FAILURE
1. Often a long history of previous episodes of breathlessness	Often produces breathlessness for the first time during middle age or after
2. Wheezing marked	Wheezing less noticeable
3. Sputum, if produced, usually thick mucoid or purulent	Sputum, if produced, usually thin and watery and often blood-stained
4. Predominantly expiratory rhonchi on chest auscultation	Predominantly basal crepitations on chest auscultation. Rhonchi, if present, are not usually confined to expiration
5. Triple rhythm (right ventricular origin) a late feature of severe bronchial asthma only	Usually additional signs of left heart failure:— *a.* Triple rhythm (left ventricular origin) *b.* Pulsus alternans
6. Usually no coexisting heart disease	Signs of underlying heart disease frequently present

INVESTIGATIONS

A chest radiograph is indicated mainly to exclude the possibility of an associated small spontaneous pneumothorax but is also helpful if the diagnosis is still in doubt. The radiological features of acute left heart failure are described in Chapter II. A chest radiograph during an attack of bronchial asthma may be normal or reveal evidence of overinflation of the lungs, i.e., increased translucency of the lung fields, horizontal ribs, low, flat, diaphragm, and a long, thin, heart shadow. Patchy collapse, resulting from plugging of the airways by thick tenacious mucus, may be seen if the attack is of some duration.

If the sputum is purulent a specimen should be collected for culture before antibiotic therapy is commenced.

A base-line E.C.G. is worth recording for, if the asthma is severe, serial tracings may provide valuable evidence of impending right ventricular strain.

MANAGEMENT

As stated previously, patients with bronchial asthma are usually only admitted to hospital when the condition is severe and conventional bronchodilator therapy has been ineffective. Vigorous treatment is essential if further deterioration is to be prevented.

1. OXYGEN

All patients with severe bronchial asthma require oxygen and this can usually be given safely in high concentration. However controlled oxygen therapy may be necessary if there is evidence of coexisting chronic airways obstruction with the possibility of an elevated arterial Pco_2. Hypercapnia may also occur as a result of severe bronchial asthma alone and the arterial oxygen and carbon dioxide tension should, if possible, be monitored in these circumstances. If this is not feasible, and there is any suspicion that the condition of the patient is deteriorating while breathing oxygen in high concentration, controlled oxygen therapy should at once be substituted. In either case, humidification of the oxygen is desirable.

2. BRONCHODILATORS

The failure of bronchial asthma to respond to a bronchodilator drug is not an indication for the prescription of combinations of such drugs in increasingly frequent dosage. Oral bronchodilators are not particularly helpful in the acute situation and there is suggestive evidence that combinations of such drugs may be responsible for the death of patients with bronchial asthma.

Although the use of subcutaneous adrenaline (0·5 ml. of 1:1000 solution) is traditional, this frequently produces a sinus tachycardia and may precipitate a more serious cardiac arrhythmia. Aminophylline, 250–500 mg. by slow intravenous injection, is the drug of choice, although this may produce nausea, vomiting, and hypotension.

3. ANTIBIOTICS

Bronchial infection is such a common precipitating factor that a broad-spectrum antibiotic is indicated even if the sputum is not obviously purulent. Ampicillin, 500 mg. 6-hourly or a combination of penicillin G 1 mega unit with streptomycin 0·5 g. intramuscularly twice daily is suitable.

4. CORTICOSTEROIDS

Until recently corticosteroids were administered only as a last resort and the condition of many patients was allowed to deteriorate seriously before they were given. It is now apparent that the prognosis of patients with severe bronchial asthma has been much improved by their early use and that very little harm is done by administering frequent large doses of hydrocortisone intravenously followed by large doses of prednisolone orally over a short period of time. The dose can be quickly reduced as the patient's condition improves.

Hydrocortisone hemisuccinate can be given initially either by repeat intravenous injection of 100 mg. or by intravenous infusion (500–1000 mg. in 1 litre of 5 per cent dextrose over 12 hours). A suitable starting dose of oral prednisolone is 80 mg. daily which can gradually be reduced over the succeeding 10 days.

5. SEDATION

Asthmatic patients often tend to be over anxious and an acute attack of breathlessness only increases their agitation. Although it might be justifiable to use a small dose of a sedative drug, e.g., chlorpromazine 50 mg. intramuscularly if the anxiety is out of proportion to the severity of the airways obstruction, the temptation to sedate patients with severe bronchial asthma (particularly with barbiturates and opiates) must be resisted for two main reasons:—

a. Restlessness in such patients is often an early indication of cerebral anoxia.

b. Sedation will further impair ventilation by depression of the respiratory centre and aggravate sputum retention by depression of the cough reflex.

6. AIDS TO EXPECTORATION

The progressive obstruction of the peripheral airways by plugs of tenacious mucus is an important and serious feature of severe prolonged bronchial asthma. If dehydration occurs the bronchial mucus becomes increasingly viscid and difficult to expectorate, and there should be no hesitation in supplementing oral with intravenous fluids if the intake of the former is inadequate.

Chest physiotherapy with supervised coughing and postural drainage is essential.

As yet, there is no convincingly effective mucolytic agent and steam inhalations have not been replaced for this purpose.

7. ASSISTED RESPIRATION AND BRONCHIAL LAVAGE

If the patient does not respond to treatment as outlined, and particularly when the danger signs (listed under CLINICAL FEATURES) of impending respiratory and circulatory failure occur, the assistance of an anaesthetist should be sought with a view to employing assisted respiration and possibly bronchial lavage. Even if the patient appears moribund, this technique is often dramatically successful.

SUMMARY

1. Hypoxaemia is common during attacks of mild bronchial asthma. Severe bronchial asthma may produce dangerous hypoxaemia, hypercapnia, and acidosis, and is a potentially lethal condition.

2. Oxygen therapy is essential for all patients with asthma and usually has no ill-effect unless the airways obstruction is so severe that respiratory failure with CO_2 retention supervenes.

3. Mucus plugging is as important a factor in the pathogenesis of variable airways obstruction as broncho-constriction, and continued efforts should be made to prevent sputum retention by vigorous chest physio-therapy, avoidance of dehydration, and humidification of the inspired oxygen.

4. Large doses of corticosteroids should be given early rather than late and less reliance placed on conventional bronchodilator drugs. A broad-spectrum antibiotic is also usually indicated.

5. Sedatives should be avoided.

6. Assisted respiration and possible bronchial lavage should not be unduly delayed if the patient's condition fails to improve, or if evidence of impending respiratory and circulatory failure appears.

Chapter VIII

ACUTE INFECTIVE EXACERBATION OF CHRONIC BRONCHITIS

ALTHOUGH often summarily dismissed by nicotine addicts as a smoker's cough, a patient suffers from chronic bronchitis when, in the absence of any localized bronchopulmonary disease, he complains of a cough productive of mucoid sputum.

Cigarette smoking and air-pollution are the most important factors concerned in the production of excessive mucoid bronchial secretion, although genetic factors and recurrent respiratory infections may play a role.

Following events such as a viral upper respiratory tract infection, a severe episode of air-pollution, chest trauma, or surgical anaesthesia, the diseased bronchi are more susceptible to secondary bacterial infection, *Hemophilus influenzae* being the organism most frequently responsible. This event is manifest clinically by a change in the appearance of the sputum from mucoid to purulent.

The breathlessness of chronic bronchitis results mainly from airways obstruction, the factors concerned in its production being:—

1. Contraction of bronchial muscle.
2. Mucosal swelling from congestion and oedema.
3. Excessive mucus in the bronchial lumen.
4. Expiratory collapse of the small airways due to a

combination of damage from recurrent infection and loss of the supporting septa if there is associated emphysema.

The first three factors are at least partially amenable to therapy but the fourth is largely irreversible.

Airways obstruction leads to uneven distribution of the inspired air throughout the lung with a consequent disturbance of ventilation/perfusion relationships. If this is severe, over-all alveolar hypoventilation with hypercapnia and hypoxaemia results. Vasoconstriction in the pulmonary vascular tree results from a reduced alveolar oxygen tension and this is probably the most important cause of pulmonary hypertension (and hence cor pulmonale) in this condition. Although widespread loss of the pulmonary vascular bed from severe emphysema must also be a factor, cor pulmonale occurs more frequently with chronic bronchitis than with emphysema.

Clinical Features

As previously stated, an acute infective exacerbation of chronic bronchitis usually results from secondary bacterial infection following a virus infection of the respiratory tract.

Characteristically the patient gives a long history of a cough productive of mucoid sputum, initially only occurring during the winter but eventually being present all the year. Breathlessness with wheezing is also a frequent complaint and there may have been previous acute infective exacerbations.

The acute illness consists of the expectoration of yellow (purulent) sputum, increasing breathlessness, fever, and general malaise.

Examination reveals an ill-looking, cyanosed, breathless patient, usually coughing large amounts of thick yellow sputum.

Physical signs may result from:—

1. The bronchitis itself.

2. Carbon dioxide retention.

3. Cor pulmonale.

1. SIGNS OF THE BRONCHITIS

Characteristic findings are:—

a. A poorly expanding, over-inflated chest which is hyperresonant on percussion.

b. Generalized expiratory and inspiratory rhonchi.

c. Coarse crepitations, due to the presence of secretions in the smaller air-passages.

2. SIGNS OF CO_2 RETENTION

As already stated, severe airways obstruction may result in alveolar hypoventilation with consequent carbon dioxide retention. The normal arterial CO_2 tension is approximately 40 mm. Hg and respiratory failure is said to be present when this level rises to over 49 mm. Hg.

Signs associated with a small elevation of arterial P_{CO_2} are:—

a. Hot hands.

b. Rapid bounding pulse.

c. Small pupils.

In addition to the above, a greater degree of CO_2 retention may cause:—

a. Engorged fundal veins.

b. Confusion or drowsiness.

c. Tremor or twitching, especially of the forearms.

Depressed tendon reflexes, extensor plantar responses, coma, and papilloedema only occur if the arterial Pco_2 is grossly elevated.

Although these signs are a useful guide to the severity of CO_2 retention, they do not remove the indication for a direct or indirect estimation of the arterial Pco_2 in these circumstances.

3. SIGNS OF COR PULMONALE

Physical signs which may be detected when the right heart is under strain are:—

  a. A prominent right ventricular impulse.

  b. Accentuation of the pulmonary second sound.

  c. A right atrial gallop, best heard at the lower end of the sternum. Evidence of associated right heart failure is indicated by:—

  a. Elevation of the jugular venous pressure.

  b. Sacral and ankle oedema.

  c. Hepatomegaly.

  d. A tricuspid pansystolic murmur.

In the event of previously impaired left ventricular function (e.g., by ischaemia, hypertension, or valvular disease), the super-added hypoxia resulting from severe airways obstruction may be sufficient to precipitate left ventricular failure. The recognition of this complication is discussed in Chapter II.

DIAGNOSIS

The diagnosis of an acute infective exacerbation of chronic bronchitis is usually easily made from the history of a cough productive of purulent sputum, associated with increasing breathlessness and wheezing, super-imposed on a background of long-standing expectoration of mucoid sputum.

Clinical examination usually serves to distinguish this condition from localized bronchopulmonary disease or bronchopneumonia but a chest radiograph should nevertheless be performed. This is also useful in excluding the possibility of an associated small spontaneous pneumothorax.

Other helpful investigations are:—

1. SPUTUM CULTURE

The result need not be awaited before antibiotic therapy is commenced but in the event of failure to respond to treatment this information is extremely valuable.

2. E.C.G.

This serves to confirm the presence of cor pulmonale and may also be helpful in indicating a previously diseased left ventricle.

3. ARTERIAL P_{CO_2}

The arterial CO_2 tension, whether measured directly on an arterial blood sample (or arterialized capillary blood) or indirectly by the rebreathing method (*see* GUIDE TO FURTHER READING for reference) is used as the indicator of the effectiveness of alveolar ventilation. A base-line estimation should be performed and oxygen therapy monitored by serial arterial P_{CO_2} measurements.

MANAGEMENT

This can best be considered under three headings:—
1. Treatment of the infection and airways obstruction.
2. Management of respiratory failure.
3. Treatment of associated heart failure.

1. TREATMENT OF THE INFECTION AND
   AIRWAYS OBSTRUCTION

This consists essentially of:—

a. Antibiotics.
b. Chest physiotherapy.
c. Bronchodilators.

a. *Antibiotic Therapy*

A broad spectrum antibiotic is indicated and either oral tetracycline or ampicillin (250–500 mg. 6-hourly) are suitable.

If a parenteral preparation is required, penicillin G 1 mega unit with streptomycin 0·5 g. intramuscularly twice daily is a useful combination. Streptomycin must be used with caution if there is any evidence of impaired renal function, and cephaloridine, up to 6·0 g. daily intramuscularly is a useful alternative, particularly when there is a history of penicillin sensitivity.

The initial régime may need to be altered if the patient's condition shows no improvement, or in the light of the result of the initial sputum culture.

b. *Chest Physiotherapy*

The prevention of sputum retention is extremely important and chest physiotherapy, consisting of regular postural drainage and the frequent encouragement of productive coughing, is essential for this purpose.

c. *Bronchodilators*

Conventional bronchodilators are not particularly helpful in the acute stage, although the slow intravenous injection of 0·25–0·5 g. aminophylline is often beneficial. Of the sympathomimetic amines, orciprenaline, 20 mg. orally 6-hourly, is one of the most useful, and this preparation can also be given by aerosol inhalation. Corticosteroids are rarely of much help and their use should be avoided if possible.

2. MANAGEMENT OF RESPIRATORY FAILURE

As previously stated, respiratory failure is defined as an elevation of the arterial Pco_2 above 49 mm. Hg.

Severe airways obstruction results in a combination of hypoxaemia and hypercapnia. As a result of the latter the respiratory centre becomes less sensitive to the stimulating effect of carbon dioxide and anoxia becomes the most important respiratory stimulus, mediated by the chemoreceptors of the carotid and aortic bodies.

Thus although the patient needs oxygen, if this is given in high concentration the sole remaining stimulus to respiration is removed, resulting in a further reduction of alveolar ventilation and a further increase in the arterial Pco_2 (*Fig. 5*).

If there are signs of CO_2 retention or the arterial Pco_2 is elevated prior to therapy, oxygen should be given continuously but in a concentration not exceeding 30 per cent. This can most easily be achieved by using a mask employing the venturi principle (e.g., Ventimask; Edinburgh mask). The condition of the patient must be carefully observed for the first hour after the commencement of controlled oxygen therapy and serial estimations of the arterial Pco_2 made if possible.

If the arterial Pco_2 continues to rise and the level of consciousness deteriorates, intravenous nikethamide 5 ml. hourly may produce some improvement, if not by stimulating respiration at least by regularly rousing the patient for a period of productive coughing.

If the patient's condition still shows no improvement, mechanical ventilation with a positive pressure respirator, in conjunction with a tracheotomy or endotracheal tube,

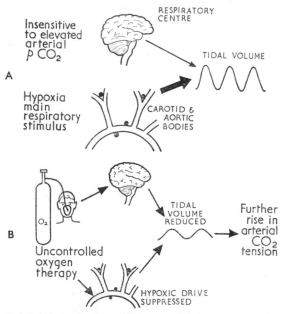

FIG. 5.—Danger of uncontrolled oxygen therapy in severe obstructive airways disease. A, Hypoxia, main respiratory stimulus, mediated by chemoreceptors of the carotid and aortic bodies. B, Uncontrolled oxygen therapy removes remaining respiratory stimulus.

will be required. Such intensive therapy is obviously not suitable for all patients and careful selection is required.

3. TREATMENT OF ASSOCIATED HEART FAILURE

By far the most important aspect of the treatment of associated heart failure is to treat the precipitating acute respiratory tract infection as outlined. Digoxin and diuretics are also indicated in conventional dosage. Morphine is contra-indicated and if this drug is inadvertently given its action can be antagonized by the intravenous injection of 5–10 mg. nalorphine, this dose being repeated as required.

Summary

1. An acute infective exacerbation of chronic bronchitis is usually the result of a super-added infection with *Haemophilus influenzae* following a virus infection of the respiratory tract.

2. The resulting airways obstruction leads to alveolar hypoventilation with consequent disturbances of the blood gases.

3. Treatment consists essentially of:—

a. A broad spectrum antibiotic.

b. Chest physiotherapy.

c. Intravenous aminophylline.

d. Controlled oxygen therapy.

4. If, despite the fact that the concentration of the inspired oxygen is carefully regulated, the arterial Pco_2 continues to rise, 5 ml. nikethamide should be given hourly by intravenous injection. If the patient's condition still shows no improvement, assisted ventilation must be considered.

5. The most important aspect of the treatment of associated heart failure is the treatment of the precipitating respiratory tract infection but digoxin and diuretics are also indicated in conventional dosage.

Chapter IX

SUBARACHNOID HAEMORRHAGE

ALTHOUGH spontaneous intracranial subarachnoid haemorrhage may occur at any age, the peak incidence is between the ages of 40 and 60 years.

The most frequent causes of this condition are:—

1. Rupture of a 'berry' aneurysm.

2. Bleeding from a vascular malformation—usually an arteriovenous angioma.

3. Arterial rupture without aneurysmal formation, usually in association with hypertension and atheromatous arterial disease.

Less common causes include rupture of a mycotic or atheromatous aneurysm, bleeding from an intra-cranial neoplasm, or as a consequence of a blood dyscrasia.

CLINICAL FEATURES

The usual mode of onset is the sudden occurrence of extremely severe headache, initially often localized to the occipital region but rapidly becoming generalized over the whole of the head. Loss of consciousness is frequent, resulting in the patient falling to the ground. Although usually short, the duration of unconsciousness may be prolonged.

Common associated features are vomiting, photophobia, and the specific complaint of discomfort on bending the neck.

Examination during the early stages of the illness reveals a distressed, vomiting, confused, and dis-orientated patient, although some of these features may occasionally be absent.

The most important physical signs, which are those of meningeal irritation as a result of the leakage of blood into the subarachnoid space, are:—

1. Neck stiffness or a complaint of discomfort when an attempt is made to flex the neck so that the chin touches the chest. Even a mild degree of neck stiffness is significant and this sign is almost invariably present in subarachnoid haemorrhage. Exceptions to this rule are:

a. If the patient is seen almost immediately after the occurrence of the haemorrhage, there may not have been time for the sign to develop.

b. Neck stiffness may sometimes be absent when the bleed has been so catastrophic that the patient is moribund.

2. Kernig's sign (spasm of the hamstring muscles when an attempt is made to extend the knee with the hip flexed to 90°) may also be positive although this is a less reliable sign of meningeal irritation than neck stiffness.

Frequent additional features are:—

a. A temporary rise of blood pressure, (although the patient may have been hypertensive prior to the haemorrhage).

b. An elevation of body temperature commonly occurs within 24 hours of the onset of the illness.

c. Transient glycosuria.

d. The rapid appearance in the optic fundus of large, bright red haemorrhages, particularly around the edge of the disc (sub-hyaloid haemorrhages).

e. Papilloedema.

Careful examination of the nervous system for the presence of focal signs is essential for, although often unreliable in accurately localizing the source of the bleeding, they may at least have some lateralizing value.

DIAGNOSIS

In practice the main problem is to distinguish subarachnoid haemorrhage from other causes of meningeal irritation, particularly meningitis. The latter is now seen comparatively infrequently in acute general medical units, most of the cases being admitted directly to a unit specializing in infectious diseases.

Although the onset of meningitis is usually less abrupt than that of subarachnoid haemorrhage, the former may occasionally develop and progress with extreme rapidity. As a result a lumbar puncture is indicated in every case where the diagnosis of subarachnoid haemorrhage is suspected. The presence of papilloedema in association with subarachnoid haemorrhage is not a contra-indication to this procedure, although it is wise to allow the C.S.F. to escape slowly.

The characteristics of the C.S.F. in subarachnoid haemorrhage are:—

1. The fluid, which is often under increased pressure, is uniformly blood-stained, best demonstrated by collecting successive samples of fluid in three small containers and comparing the amount of blood in each. If the blood is traumatic in origin the degree of blood-staining in the third container is significantly less than the first, whereas in subarachnoid haemorrhage the

sample of fluid in each of the three containers is equally blood-stained.

2. After centrifugation of the fluid the supernatant is clear but yellow (xanthochromia). This is best detected by viewing the centrifuged sample against a white background. Xanthochromia is invariably present within 24 hours after the occurrence of the haemorrhage.

3. The C.S.F. protein content is increased.

The diagnosis of the underlying lesion by clinical methods is less easy. Helpful points are:—

1. A ruptured 'berry' aneurysm may occur without prior warning, but there may be a previous history of headache and sometimes its presence causes focal neurological signs. Occasionally associated congenital anomalies are coarctation of the aorta and polycystic kidneys.

2. That the haemorrhage may have occurred from an angioma is suggested by:—

a. A previous history of strictly unilateral migraine.

b. Associated epileptic attacks.

c. Repeated episodes of subarachnoid bleeding, particularly in a young person.

d. The presence of an intracranial bruit.

3. Although a true spontaneous subarachnoid haemorrhage may occur in the elderly, the probability that the clinical picture has resulted from an intracerebral haemorrhage which has ruptured into the ventricles is usually assessed by considering the age of the patient, the severity of the neurological lesion, and the presence of hypertension and/or atheromatous arterial degeneration. The distinction between a spontaneous subarachnoid

haemorrhage, which results in the patient falling and fracturing his skull, and a subarachnoid haemorrhage of traumatic origin may be difficult or even impossible. If the patient is conscious he may remember whether the fall was preceded by a sudden headache. However this vital information is obviously not obtainable if the patient remains unconscious or is amnesic and unless the onset was witnessed the correct sequence of events remains undecided.

An E.C.G. is useful for two main reasons:—

1. To exclude the possibility that, in the event of the patient remaining unconscious or confused, the sudden collapse was the result of a myocardial infarction and the blood-stained C.S.F. traumatic in origin.

2. To aid the decision as to whether the rise of blood-pressure is a temporary event, resulting from the raised intracranial pressure, or indicative of pre-existing hypertension. (The presence of associated features of cardiovascular hypertrophy, i.e., a thrusting left ventricular impulse, a left atrial gallop, whip-cord brachial arteries, and hypertensive retinopathy, suggest that the hypertension is of some duration.)

However, it should be noted that gross E.C.G. abnormalities, simulating those of severe ischaemic heart disease, may occur as the result of the subarachnoid haemorrhage alone and considerable care is required in the interpretation of the tracing.

MANAGEMENT

If the patient is unconscious, a clear airway should be ensured and he should be nursed in the semi-prone position.

Severe headache, vomiting, and confusion are best treated by a combination of pethidine 100 mg. intramuscularly and chlorpropazine 50 mg. intramuscularly, repeated as necessary (some relief from the headache may result from the lumbar puncture). Intramuscular paraldehyde may be required if convulsions occur.

The decision concerning the advisability of cerebral arteriography in an attempt to demonstrate the nature and site of the underlying lesion prior to considering surgery, need not be taken within the first few hours of admission and consideration of this problem is beyond the scope of this book.

Summary

1. The commonest sources of subarachnoid haemorrhage are a 'berry' aneurysm, a vascular malformation, and a primary intracerebral haemorrhage which ruptures into the ventricles or subarachnoid space.

2. Sudden severe headache is the major symptom and neck stiffness the cardinal physical sign.

3. Lumbar puncture is essential to establish the diagnosis, the main features being that the C.S.F. is uniformly blood-stained and the supernatant xanthochromic after centrifugation.

4. Pethidine and chlorpromazine is the most effective drug combination for the relief of symptoms.

Chapter X

HYPERTENSIVE ENCEPHALOPATHY

As a result of the widespread use of hypotensive drugs, hypertensive encephalopathy is now one of the less common medical emergencies. The fact that the diagnosis is still made comparatively frequently can be explained by the failure to appreciate the criteria which must be fulfilled before the diagnosis can be accepted.

Since the treatment of this condition, which is a matter of urgency, differs considerably from that of some of the more common emergencies which it resembles, the recognition of true hypertensive encephalopathy when it is encountered remains of some importance.

Hypertensive encephalopathy is defined as an acute and transitory disturbance of cerebral function occurring in association with a rapid rise of diastolic blood-pressure in a patient with severe hypertension, regardless of its cause. The essential pathological features are constriction of the cerebral arterioles and cerebral oedema.

CLINICAL FEATURES

The earliest symptom is usually that of increasingly severe headache. Vomiting and disturbance of vision rapidly follow and the patient becomes progressively more drowsy. Focal cerebral disturbances may develop and eventually convulsions and coma occur.

Physical signs may be considered under three headings:

1. Those of the cerebral disturbance, indicated by convulsions, impairment of consciousness, and focal neurological signs, e.g., cortical blindness, disturbance of speech, hemiplegia, extensor plantar responses.

2. Evidence of severe hypertension, the two essential signs which must be present before the diagnosis can be made being:—

a. A diastolic blood-pressure above 140 mm. Hg.

b. Papilloedema with retinal exudates and haemorrhages.

If the hypertension is of some duration, evidence of cardiovascular hypertrophy will also be apparent.

3. Occasionally signs of the cause of the hypertension will also be evident.

DIAGNOSIS

Although headache may be caused by severe hypertension, all hypertensive patients who develop headache are not necessarily developing incipient encephalopathy and conditions such as migraine and tension headache are equally likely to be responsible. Since neck stiffness may occasionally occur in hypertensive encephalopathy, a subarachnoid haemorrhage may be suspected but can easily be distinguished by lumbar puncture (see previous chapter).

MANAGEMENT

Urgent reduction of the blood-pressure is essential and ganglion-blocking agents, although now largely of historical interest, retain their usefulness for this purpose (*Fig.* 6). As their effect is predominantly postural the head of the bed is first elevated by blocks until the bed slopes down at an angle of approximately 45 degrees.

Hexamethonium bromide is then injected intravenously at a rate of 1 mg. per minute (the blood-pressure being recorded each minute) until the diastolic pressure falls to 100 mm. Hg. At this stage intravenous

1. Parenteral hexamethonium and/or pentolinium
2. Block head of bed

1. Block foot of bed

2. I.M. Metaraminol

Frequent observation of B.P.

→ If excessive fall →

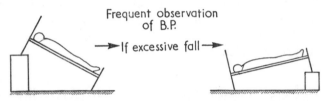

FIG. 6.—Method of using ganglion-blocking agents in hypertensive encephalopathy.

hexamethonium is replaced by the subcutaneous injection of pentolinium, the initial dose being 2·5 mg. and repeated as often as necessary to maintain the diastolic blood-pressure at around 100 mm. Hg.

Although these drugs are certainly effective hypotensive agents, their use is not always without difficulty for the following reasons:—

1. Tolerance to ganglion-blocking drugs may develop rapidly and successive doses of pentolinium may need to be considerably increased if the diastolic pressure is to be kept at a reasonable level.

2. The features of associated blockade of the parasympathetic ganglia (dry mouth, paralysis of ocular accommodation, difficulty in micturition, and constipation) are unpleasant and, if paralytic ileus occurs, may be dangerous.

3. The blood-pressure may fall too precipitately, resulting in circulatory collapse. In this event the blocks should be removed from the head of the bed and placed under the foot to place the patient in a head-down position. If the systolic pressure remains low an intramuscular injection of 5–10 mg. metaraminol should be given and repeated as often as necessary.

In view of these complications the more recently introduced hypotensive drugs, which exert their action by interrupting the transmission of the nerve-impulse from the post-ganglionic adrenergic nerve-ending to the effector cell, have been used for the treatment of hypertensive encephalopathy.

Examples of such preparations are :—

a. Guanethidine—initial dose 10–20 mg. intramuscularly, the injection being repeated after 3 hours if necessary.

b. Bethanidine—initial dose 10 mg. intravenously, repeated if necessary after 30 minutes.

(The hypotensive effect of both guanethidine and bethanidine is mainly postural and the head of the bed should be elevated as for the use of ganglion-blocking drugs.)

c. Methyldopa—initial dose 250–500 mg. intravenously repeated at 6-hourly intervals. The dose is added to 100 ml. of 5 per cent dextrose solution and infused over 30–60 minutes.

These adrenergic blockading drugs should not be used if there is a possibility that the hypertensive crisis is due to a phaeochromocytoma or associated with the administration of a monoamine oxidase inhibitor.

Once the blood-pressure has been brought under control with a parenteral preparation, this can be replaced by oral hypotensive drugs for maintenance therapy.

The occurrence of convulsions is an indication for the intramuscular administration of 10 ml. paraldehyde in addition to hypotensive agents, and the dose should be repeated half-hourly until the fits stop.

SUMMARY

1. The essential features of hypertensive encephalopathy are the sudden development of headache, vomiting, drowsiness, focal C.N.S. disturbances, convulsions, and coma in a patient with:—

a. A diastolic blood pressure of 140 mm. Hg or above.

b. Grade IV hypertensive retinopathy.

2. Urgent lowering of the blood-pressure is essential, the use of parenteral preparations of hypotensive agents being indicated.

3. In the presence of convulsions, intramuscular paraldehyde should also be given.

Chapter XI

STROKES

UNTIL comparatively recently it was thought possible by clinical methods alone to predict not only whether the cerebrovascular disturbance responsible for an acute neurological deficit was due either to a cerebral thrombosis, haemorrhage, or embolic episode, but also the site of the vascular pathology with reasonable accuracy.

The falsity of these assumptions has been amply demonstrated by both post-mortem studies and cerebral angiography in patients with strokes, and in particular the concept of cerebral thrombosis has now been replaced by that of 'non-embolic infarction'. Atheromatous occlusive disease remains the predominant arterial lesion but often no vascular occlusion can be demonstrated by arteriography, and atheroma of the extra-cranial portions of the carotid and vertebral arteries may be responsible for stroke causation.

A sudden vascular disturbance may result in damage to any part of the brain but by far the most frequent form of stroke presentation is the sudden development of a hemiplegia of varying severity. The practical problems when dealing with such patients are :—

1. To decide, if possible, the nature of the cerebro-vascular disturbance.

2. To differentiate vascular from non-vascular causes of an acute neurological deficit.

3. To decide whether any specific therapeutic measures are indicated.

THE UNDERLYING CEREBROVASCULAR DISTURBANCE

As already stated, it is now realized that it is impossible to diagnose the underlying vascular pathology of a stroke with absolute certainty by clinical methods alone. Nevertheless, certain features enable a shrewd guess to be made as to whether cerebral haemorrhage, embolism, or non-embolic infarction is responsible.

1. CEREBRAL HAEMORRHAGE

The onset is usually sudden with headache and vomiting and frequently loss of consciousness. Hypertension is an almost invariable associated feature. The condition of the patient often deteriorates rapidly and the neural structures involved are outside the distribution of a single artery.

2. CEREBRAL EMBOLISM

Again the stroke is of sudden onset, the patient often relatively young and a potential source of the embolus is present (commonly atrial fibrillation in association with mitral stenosis or endocardial thrombus following a myocardial infarction). Loss of consciousness is unusual, improvement tends to be fairly rapid, and the neural structures involved lie within the territory of a single artery.

3. NON-EMBOLIC INFARCTION

Although now the commonest cause of strokes, diagnosis is essentially a matter of exclusion, the features of embolism and haemorrhage being absent. The patient is frequently past middleage and there may be clinical

Table III.—Features which aid the Differentiation between Cerebral Haemorrhage, Embolism, and Non-embolic Infarction

	Cerebral Haemorrhage	Cerebral Embolism	Non-embolic Infarction
Clinical features	Explosive onset with headache and vomiting. Loss of consciousness usual. Rapid deterioration. Associated hypertension. Neural structures involved outside distribution of a single artery	Sudden onset. Patient often relatively young. Consciousness rarely lost. Potential source of embolus apparent. Tendency to rapid recovery. Neural structures involved within territory of a single artery	Patient past middle age. No source of emboli apparent. Occasionally evidence of atheromatous disease of neck arteries
C.S.F.	Frequently blood-stained and under increased pressure	Clear fluid, normal pressure	Clear fluid, normal pressure
Echoencephalogram	Mid-line structures may be displaced from the onset	No displacement of mid-line structures in the early stages	No displacement of mid-line structures in the early stages

evidence of atheromatous degeneration of the major arteries in the neck (unequal carotid pulses or a bruit over the carotid or vertebral arteries).

These features, together with the typical lumbar puncture and echoencephalographic findings, are summarized in *Table III*.

DIAGNOSIS

1. UNCOMMON CAUSES OF 'STROKES'

Although atheromatous arterial occlusive disease is the major cause of non-embolic infarction, other possibilities are meningovascular syphilis, polycythaemia, or a form of arteritis. A painless myocardial infarction may occasionally be responsible and a non-embolic infarct may also follow a few hours or days after an acute gastro-intestinal haemorrhage (suggesting that the cause is some change in the blood constituents rather than the transient hypotension).

Sub-acute bacterial endocarditis should always be considered if there is no other obvious source of a cerebral embolus and a blood culture is mandatory if a sudden stroke occurs in a patient with a low-grade fever and a cardiac murmur.

Meningism is usually the outstanding feature of a ruptured cerebral aneurysm but occasionally the focal neurological deficit may be predominant.

2. AIDS TO THE DIFFERENTIATION BETWEEN CEREBRAL HAEMORRHAGE, EMBOLISM, AND NON-EMBOLIC INFARCTION

a. *Lumbar Puncture*

Uniformly blood-stained C.S.F. under increased pressure occurs both in a primary intracerebral haemorrhage, which has ruptured into the ventricle, and as a result of bleeding from a 'berry' aneurysm or arterio-venous malformation. Unfortunately approximately 20 per cent of patients who have suffered a cerebral haemorrhage do not have blood-stained C.S.F., although the C.S.F. pressure is usually elevated. Blood-staining of the C.S.F. is not usually a feature of either cerebral embolism or non-embolic infarction.

b. *Echoencephalography*

Brain scanning with ultra sound is an easy, painless procedure which can be done immediately after admission and is well within the scope of a pre-registration house-physician. The apparatus is not yet generally available but its usefulness is increasingly being appreciated. Its main application is to demonstrate whether any shift of the mid-line structures has occurred. If this feature is observed in the early stages of the illness, a cerebral haemorrhage (or any other intracranial space-occupying lesion) is the most likely explanation. A shift of the mid-line structures detected in the later stages of the illness is equally likely to be due to oedema resulting from a cerebral embolus or a non-embolic infarct.

c. *Cerebral Arteriography*

Although an invaluable aid to the differential diagnosis of strokes in selected patients, this is rarely indicated as an emergency procedure.

3. CONDITIONS WHICH MAY MIMIC STROKES

Although the diagnosis of a stroke rarely causes much difficulty, cerebral tumours (primary or secondary) may occasionally cause an acute neurological deficit, usually either as a result of haemorrhage into a cystic or necrotic lesion or pressure from the tumour causing a venous infarction.

Features which suggest that a tumour might be responsible for the occurrence of a sudden hemiplegia are:—

a. The presence of papilloedema in the early stages of the illness.

b. High C.S.F. protein content (in the absence of blood-staining).

c. Shift of the mid-line structures of the brain as demonstrated by echoencephalography.

d. Evidence of a primary tumour elsewhere in the body.

In view of the possibility of surgical cure of a subdural haematoma, this condition should always be considered even when there is no history of a preceding head injury. If the severity of the hemiplegia is greater than the disturbance of consciousness, a sub-dural collection is unlikely but if there is any doubt, the patient should be referred for full neurosurgical investigation.

It may occasionally be difficult to decide whether a stroke, which is first observed after a fall, is due to the consequences of cerebral trauma or the stroke responsible for the fall. In practice, the correct sequence is of little importance initially since if there is external or radiographic evidence of a head injury, the case must be managed as such for, regardless of the cause of the fall, the patient will be liable to all the possible complications.

From the above discussion it can be seen that it is advisable to institute the following investigations as soon as possible after a patient with a stroke has been admitted to hospital:—

1. Radiograph of chest and skull.
2. Full blood-count and E.S.R.
3. Blood Wassermann reaction.
4. E.C.G.
5. Lumbar puncture (except in the presence of gross papilloedema).
6. Echoencephalography (if available).

Although these investigations may not be indicated in every case (e.g., in an elderly patient with a terminal cerebrovascular episode) their use will lessen the chance of a remediable lesion being mistaken for the consequence of degenerative arterial disease.

MANAGEMENT

A severe hemiplegia is a catastrophic occurrence in any patient and many methods of improving cerebral blood-flow have been tried in an attempt to limit the neuronal damage. Unfortunately none have been shown to be convincingly effective if the stroke is fully developed at the time of admission.

If the patient is unconscious the first essential is to ensure a clear airway and the patient is subsequently nursed in the semi-prone position. Routine care of the unconscious patient should then be instituted, particular attention being payed to the state of hydration, care of the skin, and the prevention of urinary incontinence, with an indwelling catheter in female patients and the use of Paul's tubing in males. Chest physiotherapy and regular passive movement of the paralysed limbs should be started from the outset.

ANTICOAGULANTS

The indications for the use of anticoagulants in cerebrovascular disease are few and the contra-indications many. The latter are:—

1. General, i.e., the presence of a peptic ulcer, hepatic disease, renal failure, or a haemorrhagic tendency.

2. The presence of uncontrolled hypertension.

3. Any evidence to suggest that either a previous or the present cerebrovascular episode is due to cerebral haemorrhage.

Anticoagulants are of no benefit in a fully developed stroke as a result of non-embolic infarction. Situations where this form of therapy is indicated are:—

1. During the acute stage of cerebral embolism and also to reduce the incidence of further embolic episodes.

2. To limit the progression of a stroke when the clinical picture is still evolving at the time of admission.

The standard method of anticoagulant administration is adopted, i.e., an intravenous infusion of heparin for the first 36–48 hours (40,000 units of heparin being added to 1 litre of 5 per cent dextrose solution and infused over 24 hours), warfarin being commenced at the same time (initial dose 40 mg. followed by 5 mg. 48 hours later, subsequent doses being regulated by serial estimations of the prothrombin time).

It must be stressed that in view of the difficulty of distinguishing cerebral haemorrhage from embolic or non-embolic infarction, even after full investigation, this form of therapy is potentially hazardous.

SURGERY

With the following two exceptions, this has little to offer:—

1. When an intracerebral haematoma continues to expand by attracting fluid into itself and thus acts as a progressive space-occupying lesion.

2. Spontaneous haemorrhage into the cerebellum. Although this may be suspected clinically, diagnosis is difficult and neuroradiological investigations are essential.

Transient Strokes

It occasionally happens that the neurological deficit of a patient, who is referred for admission on the basis of having suffered a stroke, has either improved before arrival at hospital or does so shortly afterwards.

Such episodes are usually the result of transient ischaemia occurring either in the carotid or vertebro-basilar territory, although alternative non-vascular causes, such as focal epilepsy, must also be considered.

The commonest cause of transient ischaemic episodes, which are often recurrent, is temporary plugging of a distal artery by platelet or clot emboli arising from ulcerated atheromatous plaques in the carotid or vertebral arteries. The investigation and treatment (by anticoagulants or surgery of the great vessels) of such attacks is not a medical emergency but nevertheless should not be unduly delayed, for a transient stroke may herald the occurrence of a much more severe cerebro-vascular disturbance.

It should be noted that there are many causes of transient ischaemic episodes other than micro-embolization

Table IV.—Causes of Transient Ischaemic Episodes

Cause	Helpful Diagnostic Features
Hypotensive episode e.g. myocardial infarction or paroxysmal arrhythmia	History of chest pain or palpitations E.C.G. abnormalities
Paroxysmal hypertension	Blood-pressure elevated during attack
Transient occlusion of the vertebral arteries in association with degenerative disease of the cervical spine	Attacks precipitated by neck extension or rotation. Radiograph cervical spine
Severe anaemia or polycythaemia	Appearance of mucosae. Blood-count
Subclavian steal, i.e., occlusion of the subclavian artery proximal to the origin of the vertebral so that the direction of vertebral blood-flow is reversed	Attacks associated with exerting the arms. Blood-pressure difference between the two arms
Recurrent cerebral emboli associated with rheumatic heart disease	Atrial fibrillation or other arrhythmia. Mitral stenosis
Migraine	Severe unilateral headache. History of previous similar headaches with typical migraine aura

and these are summarized, together with helpful diagnostic points, in *Table IV.*

Summary

1. The differentiation between cerebral haemorrhage, embolism, and non-embolic infarction may be extremely difficult, even after full investigation.

2. Although atheromatous arterial disease is the commonest cause of strokes, the less frequent causes should always be considered when dealing with an acutely hemiplegic patient.

3. The possibility of a cerebral tumour or a sub-dural haematoma presenting as an acute neurological deficit must always be remembered.

4. Apart from anticoagulant therapy, which is indicated only occasionally, and surgery which is indicated even less frequently, there is no specific treatment.

5. The main importance of transient ischaemic episodes, due to micro-embolization from ulcerated atheromatous plaques in the carotid or vertebral arteries, is that they may herald a major stroke.

Chapter XII

TRANSIENT UNCONSCIOUSNESS

TEMPORARY loss of consciousness in an ambulant patient usually results in him being brought to the casualty department of the nearest hospital. Admission to the medical ward for a period of observation and investigation usually follows unless the cause of the 'black-out', (used to imply loss of consciousness rather than loss of vision) is obvious and no immediate action is judged to be necessary.

The fundamental causes of most episodes of transient unconsciousness are:—

A. Temporary ischaemia of the brain-stem as a result of systemic arterial hypotension (syncope).

B. Hypoglycaemia (blood-glucose below 40 mg./ 100 ml.).

C. Epilepsy.

Also feigned unconsciousness may occasionally be encountered.

The characteristic features of each of these causes of transient loss of consciousness are summarized in *Table V.*

The diagnosis of the cause of an unconscious episode largely depends on an accurate account of the circumstances and events leading up to the attack, and the appearance of the patient both during and immediately after the episode. It is thus essential when dealing with

	SYNCOPE	HYPOGLYCAEMIA	EPILEPSY	FEIGNED UNCONSCIOUSNESS
Events and symptoms preceding unconscious episode	Simple fainting attack usually preceded by nausea and sweating associated with feeling of weakness and lightheadedness. May be an obvious precipitating factor	Early symptoms are headache, irritability, sweating, lack of concentration, irrational or aggressive behaviour. May be spontaneous or result from a missed meal, excessive physical exertion or a wrong dose of insulin in a diabetic patient	May be an epileptic aura (frequently an unpleasant sensation arising in the epigastrium) but often no warning	Usually occurs in a characteristic type of patient. Purpose for the attack normally apparent
Appearance while unconscious	Pale and sweaty with low blood pressure. Pulse slow during simple fainting attack but may be fast or irregular if there is an organic cause. Convulsive movements and incontinence of urine or faeces infrequent	Warm, sweaty skin. Full volume pulse. Dilated pupils. Plantars often extensor and may be other focal C.N.S. signs. Convulsions infrequent but may occur if hypoglycaemia profound	Sudden fall may result in injury. Tonic followed by clonic phase (tongue biting, foaming at the mouth, and incontinence may occur during latter). Plantars often extensor and corneal and tendon reflexes may be absent	Whether motionless or struggling violently, patient resists attempts to open eyes, tendon reflexes unchanged, and plantars flexor. Usually dramatic response to painful stimuli. Physical injury as a result of fall or struggling movements very uncommon
Following period of unconsciousness	Recumbency usually results in rapid return of consciousness. Drowsiness or confusion uncommon after a syncopal attack	Administration of glucose usually results in rapid return of consciousness	Often drowsy and confused and usually sleep for several hours. May be period of post-epileptic automatism	Not of diagnostic importance

this problem to obtain a detailed description of these events from any available witnesses and such persons should always be interviewed by the receiving house-physician before they leave the hospital.

A. Syncope

Regardless of the cause, the characteristics of a syncopal attack are that during the episode the patient lies still. The skin is pale and sweaty and the blood-pressure low. Convulsive movements and incontinence of urine or faeces are unusual. When recumbent the period of unconsciousness is usually short and rapid recovery is the rule.

The commonest form of syncope is probably the *simple uncomplicated faint*, due either to instability or inefficiency of the vasomotor centre. Such attacks are commonly precipitated by emotional shock, pain, exhaustion, recent illness, a hot atmosphere, or a long period of standing in the same position. Frequent premonitory symptoms are a feeling of weakness, nausea, sweating, and lightheadedness, and the patient usually remembers falling. A simple faint can not occur when the patient is recumbent and is usually associated with marked bradycardia.

Postural hypotension, induced by a sudden change from the lying to the standing position, may occasionally be severe enough to cause fainting and is frequently iatrogenic, many hypotensive drugs possessing this undesirable side-effect. The sudden vasodilatation pro-duced by trinitrin is occasionally responsible for a patient with ischaemic heart disease fainting, when this drug is used for the relief of anginal pain.

Transient hypotension may also result from a sudden fall in cardiac output, and disorders of the heart which may be responsible for syncopal attacks are:—

1. Any condition where there is central circulatory obstruction, i.e., aortic stenosis, pulmonary stenosis, pulmonary hypertension, and ball-valve obstruction of the mitral valve.

2. Sudden changes of rhythm.

3. Heart block (Stokes-Adams attacks—due to the sudden development of a ventricular arrhythmia or asystole).

4. Myocardial infarction.

The cause of cardiogenic syncope can usually be decided by a combination of careful physical examination and electrocardiography.

Forms of *reflex syncope* are:—

1. *Cough Syncope.*—Although a syncopal attack may follow a paroxysm of coughing, all unconscious attacks which follow such an event are not necessarily syncopal and care should be taken to exclude an underlying focal cerebral lesion.

2. *Carotid Sinus Syncope.*—This classically occurs in a middle-aged or elderly patient who, while wearing a tight collar, falls unconscious after turning the head.

3. *Micturition Syncope.*—A syncopal attack may occur as a result of a male with lower urinary tract obstruction straining excessively to pass urine, usually in the middle of the night.

Syncopal attacks may also result from:—

1. Atheromatous occlusive disease of the carotid and vertebral arteries, so that the cerebral blood-flow is more than usually dependent on an adequate perfusion pressure. In these circumstances even minor changes in cardiac output may cause cerebral ischaemia.

2. Sudden blood-loss, e.g., a gastro-intestinal haemorrhage may result in a patient being brought to the casualty department after a syncopal attack before any blood is either vomited or passed as a melaena stool.

Patients with chronic anaemia are also more liable to syncopal attacks.

INVESTIGATIONS AND MANAGEMENT

Although the cause of a syncopal attack can usually be ascertained by a careful history and physical examination, a blood-count, chest film, and E.C.G. are often helpful.

The attack itself is treated by laying the patient flat; this is usually all that is necessary and consciousness quickly returns.

Stokes-Adams attacks are potentially lethal and if consciousness does not return within a few seconds, a few sharp blows should be delivered to the sternum. If recovery still does not occur, external cardiac massage and assisted respiration must be commenced and an electrocardiograph tracing obtained. Electrical defibrillation should abolish ventricular arrhythmias and may be sufficient to restart the heart beating if it is in asystole. In the latter event, 0·5 ml. of 1:1000 adrenaline may be given intramuscularly or intravenously. The use of an electrical pacemaker may be necessary if ventricular asystole is persistent.

Other causes of syncopal episodes should be treated whenever possible.

B. HYPOGLYCAEMIA

This problem, which is most frequently encountered in diabetic patients receiving insulin therapy, is discussed in detail in Chapter XVI.

Spontaneous hypoglycaemia occasionally occurs, by far the most important cause being an insulin-secreting tumour of the pancreas. This diagnosis is suggested by the tendency for the unconscious attack to occur after a prolonged period of starvation, associated profuse sweating, and prompt relief after the administration of glucose. A blood sample should be taken during the period of unconsciousness for estimation of the glucose content and if this is always done when the cause of transient loss of consciousness is not apparent, the chances of making an erroneous diagnosis will be reduced. If the possibility of an insulin-secreting tumour is raised by the finding of a low blood-glucose, more specific biochemical investigations are obviously indicated.

Reactive hypoglycaemia is usually suggested by the occurrence of hypoglycaemic symptoms shortly after a large carbohydrate meal.

C. EPILEPSY

The features of a major epileptic attack are well known. Often there is a recognizable epileptic aura, most commonly taking the form of an unpleasant epigastric sensation spreading up to the head. The patient may then utter a cry and fall heavily to the ground, frequently sustaining physical injury. The tonic phase, when all the muscles are in spasm and the patient cyanosed, is followed by the clonic phase, during which regular convulsive movements of the trunk, limbs, jaws, and tongue occur. Foaming at the mouth, tongue-biting, and incontinence of urine and faeces commonly occur at this stage.

The patient then usually regains consciousness within a few minutes but may remain unconscious for an hour or more. When consciousness does return the patient is drowsy, often confused, frequently complains of headache, and tends to fall asleep quickly.

The plantar responses are frequently extensor during the attack and other focal neurological signs, which are often transient, may also be apparent.

MANAGEMENT

The patient rarely suffers any physical harm as a result of a major epileptic convulsion if a clear airway is ensured, a padded gag placed between the teeth, and the patient removed from possible contact with neighbouring objects.

Frequently the patient will be known to suffer from epilepsy and after a short period of observation together with any necessary adjustment of the régime of anticonvulsant drugs, he can be discharged home.

If the convulsion is the first such episode in an adult patient, the cause should be determined if possible, full neurological investigation often being required for this purpose. Fits may occur as the result of barbiturate withdrawal from an addict and this possibility must always be remembered when considering the possible causes of convulsions of late onset.

D. Feigned Unconsciousness

Although this is mainly a problem for the casualty officer, the house-physician is often requested to see unconscious patients in the casualty department, and advise on their management.

Feigned unconsciousness is likely to be encountered in three types of patient:—

1. Hysterical females.
2. Genuine epileptics who also have hysterical fits.
3. Vagrant, unemployed persons who are seeking food and accommodation.

Most hysterical fits or blackouts, for which there is always a purpose, are easy to diagnose if they are witnessed. There is no orderly sequence of events and consciousness is not genuinely lost. The patient rarely injures herself as a result of falling and there is no incontinence or tongue-biting. The limb movements are not a series of regular jerks but wild and struggling and are usually aggravated if any attempt is made at physical restraint. Also, in contrast to a genuine epileptic fit, attempts to open the eyes are met with by tightly shutting the lids, the tendon jerks are normal, and the plantar responses flexor.

Additional hysterical fits produced by a genuine epileptic patient are much more difficult to diagnose with certainty but careful observation of an unconscious episode usually enables the distinction to be made.

Feigned unconsciousness is usually easy to recognize in a vagrant, unemployed person who is brought into the casualty department having apparently 'collapsed' in the street. Again physical signs are lacking and attempts to open the eyelids are resisted. Such patients are usually unresponsive to pin-prick but more painful stimuli, such as supra-orbital pressure, frequently have a rousing effect. If more unpleasant methods are employed in an attempt to terminate the act, care should be taken that the examiner is out of striking distance of the patient who often tends to be rather aggressive under these circumstances.

STATUS EPILEPTICUS

Although by definition the unconsciousness in this condition is not transient, it is convenient to include a discussion of status epilepticus at this stage. This term is used to describe the occurrence of fits in quick succession, without the patient regaining consciousness between each. Recognition of this potentially lethal emergency presents no problems.

Paraldehyde 10 ml. intramuscularly (preferably given as two 5 ml. injections at different sites) which can be repeated every 30 minutes while the fits continue, is usually successful.

Alternative régimes which may be employed in preference to paraldehyde, or in the event of the latter drug being unsuccessful in controlling the convulsions, are:—

1. An intravenous injection of 250 mg. (5 ml.) phenytoin at a rate of 1 ml. per minute. This may need to be repeated after 30 minutes if the fits continue and the condition subsequently controlled by repeated injection of 100 mg. intramuscularly.

2. The slow intravenous injection of diazepam in 10 mg. doses until either control is achieved or a total of 40–50 mg. has been given over 1–2 hours.

3. A slow intravenous injection or a continuous intravenous infusion of a short-acting barbiturate such as thiopentone or methohexitone. This technique requires the ready availability of an anaesthetist who can assist ventilation if significant respiratory depression should occur.

Once the emergency has been dealt with, the cause of the status epilepticus should be ascertained if possible, by far the most common precipitant being the sudden cessation of regular anticonvulsant medication.

SUMMARY

1. A witnessed account of the appearance of the patient prior to and during the period of unconsciousness is an invaluable aid to discovering the cause of the disorder.

2. The three basic causes of transient attacks of unconsciousness are:—

a. Transient cerebral ischaemia (syncope).

b. Hypoglycaemia.

c. Epilepsy.

3. Each of these fundamental disturbances may themselves be due to a number of causes, the diagnosis of the relevant one being of vital importance.

4. Feigned unconsciousness occasionally occurs but its recognition is usually comparatively easy.

Chapter XIII

DRUG OVERDOSAGE

SELF-ADMINISTERED overdosage of drugs is responsible for an increasing number of medical emergency admissions to hospital. Although such poisoning in children is usually accidental, when it occurs in adults it is almost invariably deliberate and is usually done either in an effort to commit suicide or as a desperate impulsive gesture to attract attention or help as a means of escaping from an awkward or unpleasant environmental situation.

Regardless of the motivation behind the drug overdosage, all patients who have taken an excess of drugs, whether or not they are physically ill as a result, should be admitted to hospital for at least a short period of observation. By following this rule, and also obtaining a psychiatric assessment of each patient, the risk of mistaking a genuine suicidal attempt in a seriously depressed patient for an impulsive gesture made to attract sympathy and attention, can be considerably reduced.

As much information as possible should be obtained from all available sources at the time of the patient's admission. The next-of-kin or a close relative should be asked both about previous psychiatric illnesses and the present mental state. Details of previous physical illnesses are also required for such information may have considerable influence on the management of a seriously poisoned patient (*see below*). This second-hand information is obviously necessary if the patient's level of consciousness is impaired but even if he is fully conscious, details which he volunteers in this particular situation may be quite unreliable and certainly need to be checked.

The person who discovers the patient should be asked about the circumstances at the time, e.g., whether an empty bottle (or bottles) were close at hand and whether a suicide note had been written. Other sources for this type of information are the police, if they have been involved, or a member of the ambulance crew.

The identity of the drug (or drugs) taken must be established as soon as possible. The drug containers may be labelled or it may be possible to recognize the remaining tablets on sight. If any difficulty is experienced the doctor who prescribed the drugs or the chemist who made up the prescription should be contacted. Another possibility if a sample of the drug is available, is the use of a tablet and capsule identification guide which should be available in all casualty departments.

With the ever increasing number of drugs in circulation, it is perhaps surprising that barbiturates and salicylates are still the most favoured preparations for self-administered drug overdosage and the management of barbiturate and salicylate intoxication will be discussed in detail.

Information concerning the possible effects and management of overdosage with other drugs can usually be obtained by reference to a suitable book dealing with this problem (*see* GUIDE TO FURTHER READING) or by contacting any of the Poisons Information Centres in Great Britain which offer a round-the-clock telephone service. These centres are at present located in London, Leeds, Cardiff, Newcastle upon Tyne, Edinburgh, and Manchester and their respective telephone numbers (Extension—Poisons Information) are as follows:—

01–HOP–7600
0532–32799
0222–33101
0632–25131
031–FOU–2477
061–CHE–2254

A. BARBITURATE INTOXICATION

The barbiturates are essentially depressants of the central nervous system and their effect (the degree of which depends on the dose taken, the duration of action of the drug, the time which has elapsed after its ingestion, whether the patient is accustomed to taking barbiturates, co-incidental renal disease, etc.) is a depression of all forms of nervous activity. This is manifest by:—

1. Depression of the level of consciousness, ranging from drowsiness to deep coma, where there is no response to maximal painful stimulation.

2. Depression of the respiratory centre, the respiratory rate being slowed and the depth of respiration reduced. Severe barbiturate poisoning may cause respiratory failure.

3. Depression of the activity of the vasomotor centre, the most important effect being loss of venous tone with a consequent expansion of the capacity of the vascular system. Since the blood-volume remains unchanged, or is reduced if there is accompanying dehydration, this results in systemic hypotension, tachycardia, and a diminished arterial pulse volume.

4. Depression of the temperature-regulating mechanism with a consequent fall in body temperature.

5. Depression of other reflex activity, i.e., sluggish or absent pupillary, corneal, and tendon reflexes.

Thus the appearance of a patient who has taken an overdose of barbiturates may vary from being drowsy but otherwise normal to being deeply comatose and cyanosed with a low body temperature, pale, cold peripheries, hypotension, a fast, poor volume pulse, extremely shallow slow respirations, and an absence of all reflex activity.

DIAGNOSIS

Although in theory, all other causes of impairment of consciousness must be considered, in practice the diagnosis of barbiturate overdosage is rarely difficult and can usually be made clinically by a consideration of the clinical features and the circumstantial evidence of drug overdosage.

Confirmation is obtained by measuring the amount of barbiturate in the serum but although rapid methods for this estimation are now available, the conventional method is time consuming and treatment usually needs to be instituted before the result is obtained.

The serum barbiturate level depends on many factors but figures which may be expected in varying degrees of poisoning, with either short- or long-acting barbiturate preparations are given in *Table VI*. However it should be noted that there is frequently little correlation between the severity of poisoning as judged clinically and the serum barbiturate level. Thus the value of this estimation is essentially diagnostic rather than as an aid to therapy.

Table VI.—SERUM BARBITURATE LEVELS (MG. BARBITURATE PER 100 ML.) FOUND IN VARYING DEGREES OF BARBITURATE INTOXICATION

	SEVERITY OF INTOXICATION		
	Mild	Moderately severe	Dangerous
Short-acting barbiturates (e.g., quinalbarbitone, cyclobarbitone)	1·0–2·0	3·0–4·0	4·0 or over
Intermediate-acting barbiturates (e.g., amylobarbitone, pentobarbitone)	1·7–4·2	6·0	7·0 or over
Long-acting barbiturates (e.g., phenobarbitone)	5·0–8·0	9·0	10·0 or over

MANAGEMENT

Most cases of barbiturate intoxication recover without specific treatment and can be discharged from hospital after a short period of observation if there is no underlying psychiatric condition which requires treatment, and when any necessary after-care has been arranged.

If the patient is deeply unconscious the first essential is to establish a clear airway. This can often be achieved by removing secretions and other foreign material from the oropharynx, turning the patient into the semi-prone position and inserting an oropharyngeal airway to assist in keeping the tongue away from the posterior pharyngeal wall. Oxygen can be given in high concentration via a face mask.

With more severe respiratory depression, an endo-trachcal tube should immediately be inserted. This has the great advantage of permitting secretions to be aspirated from the trachea and major bronchi and also enables assisted ventilation with a mechanical ventilator to be commenced at any time. The latter should be started without hesitation if the patient is cyanosed with feeble spontaneous respirations or if the blood gases are seriously disturbed.

After an unobstructed airway has been ensured, the question of gastric lavage must be considered. There is little to be gained by this procedure if over 4 hours have elapsed between the time of barbiturate ingestion and arrival at hospital. If less than 4 hours have elapsed, gastric lavage is worthwhile but should only be done in an unconscious patient if a cuffed endo-tracheal tube is in situ to prevent the inhalation of gastric washings.

Systemic hypotension often responds to elevating the foot of the bed but if the systolic pressure remains below 90 mm. Hg, an intramuscular injection of 5 mg. metaraminol should be given and repeated if necessary. If the blood-pressure remains low, the increased capacity of the vascular bed must be filled by increasing the blood-volume. This can be achieved by either blood transfusion or the infusion of plasma or dextran, the amount required being judged by frequent observation of the pulse-rate and blood-pressure or by monitoring the central venous pressure.

Fluid and electrolyte balance must be maintained (the intravenous route is easiest for this purpose), bladder catheterization may be necessary, and routine nursing care of the unconscious patient must be instituted.

Forced diuresis, peritoneal dialysis, and haemo-dialysis have all been used to shorten the period of unconsciousness following severe barbiturate overdosage and thus reduce the risk of complications. Forced diuresis and peritoneal dialysis are both methods which can be employed in non-specialist units, but the former is probably the easiest in practice and the technique will be discussed in detail. It should be noted that forced diuresis is not indicated in all cases of barbiturate intoxication and should only be used if the poisoning is clinically judged to be severe.

Forced Diuresis

This consists essentially of the intravenous administration of large volumes of fluid, thus increasing the urine flow and hence the rate of drug elimination (*Fig.* 7A, B). The latter is further increased by alkalinization of the urine, for barbiturates are weak acids and the rate of phenobarbitone excretion in particular is considerably increased by this method. Forced diuresis is a potentially dangerous technique and its use is conditional on there being:—

1. No history of renal or cardiac disease.

2. A satisfactory blood-pressure (systolic level of greater than 90 mm. Hg).

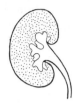

1.
Normal renal
function

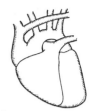

2.
No evidence of
cardiac disease

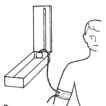

3.
Systolic B.P. of at
least 90mm. of Hg

A

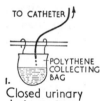

TO CATHETER

POLYTHENE
COLLECTING
BAG

1.
Closed urinary
drainage to en-
able accurate
assessment of
urinary output

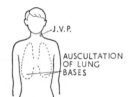

J.V.P.

AUSCULTATION
OF LUNG
BASES

2.
Frequent examination
to detect signs of
fluid overload

3.
Adequate
supervision of fast
– running infusion

B

Fig. 7.—A, Pre-requisites for forced diuresis. B, Precautions during
forced diuresis.

3. No abnormality in the urine and a normal blood-
urea.

4. Trained staff available to supervise the rapid
intravenous infusion.

If there is no contra-indication, and there is clinical evidence of severe barbiturate intoxication, the diuresis is established as follows:—

1. The bladder must be catheterized and closed urinary drainage established so that an accurate record of the urine output is available.

2. An intravenous infusion is set up and the following infused in rotation:—

> 500 ml. 5 per cent dextrose and 50 mEq. sodium bicarbonate over 30 min.
>
> 500 ml. 5 per cent dextrose and 25 mEq. potassium chloride over 30 min.
>
> 500 ml. normal saline over 30 min.

This sequence is then repeated for the next 90-minute period, after which the infusion rate is reduced to 500 ml. per hour, although the same rotation of fluids is employed.

3. A diuretic is administered, 40 mg. frusemide intravenously usually being satisfactory and as effective as ethacrynic acid or the infusion of mannitol.

As the patient's condition improves, so the rate of fluid infusion can be reduced.

If the condition of the patient deteriorates despite a forced diuresis, or if this technique cannot be employed because of persistent hypotension or the presence of renal or cardiac disease, haemodialysis is indicated.

Prophylactic antibiotics should not be given as a routine but reserved for use when there is clinical or radiological evidence of a chest infection or if there is a possibility of the patient having inhaled vomit.

Central stimulants, e.g., bemegride or nikethamide, have no place in the management of barbiturate intoxication.

B. Salicylate Intoxication

The clinical features of salicylate intoxication are dizziness, excitability, tinnitus, dimness of vision, nausea and vomiting, and over-breathing. There is usually a tachycardia but the pulse volume is good. Depression of the level of consciousness is a late feature of salicylate poisoning and therefore its absence does not necessarily mean that the patient is not seriously poisoned. When unconsciousness does occur, usually only a short period elapses before circulatory collapse and death ensues.

DIAGNOSIS

Again clinical diagnosis is comparatively easy although the condition could conceivably be confused with diabetic coma in view of the over-breathing and keto-nuria. The resemblance is usually, however, only superficial and their distinction in practice rarely causes any difficulty.

Confirmation of the diagnosis is obtained by measuring the serum salicylate level which in cases of intoxication is usually greater than 50 mg. per 100 ml.

MANAGEMENT

Gastric lavage is well worthwhile in patients who have taken an overdose of salicylates regardless of the time interval between ingestion of the drug and arrival at hospital, for salicylates are frequently retained in the stomach for many hours. Also the patient is usually conscious so that the risk of inhalation of gastric contents does not arise.

Mild cases can often be treated by ensuring a high oral intake of fluids but if there is clinical evidence of severe salicylism, or if the serum salicylate value is high, the technique of forced diuresis should be employed. The régime and its contra-indications are as for barbiturate intoxication except that bicarbonate should *not* be added to the infusion fluid as the major acid-base disturbance resulting from salicylate intoxication is a respiratory alkalosis which persists throughout the course of the illness. Infusion of bicarbonate may dangerously increase this alkalosis and unless facilities are available to confirm that the pH of the arterial blood is normal, the technique of forced diuresis should be employed without the addition of alkali.

If the serum salicylate level is over 100 mg./100 ml., if the patient is unconscious, or if there is evidence of circulatory collapse or that forced diuresis has been ineffective, haemodialysis is almost certainly indicated.

The ingestion of large doses of aspirin occasionally causes bleeding from the gastric mucosa which may be severe enough to require blood transfusion. If hypoprothrombinaemia, which is an uncommon complication of salicylate intoxication, should occur, an intramuscular injection of 10 mg. phytomenadione should be given.

SUMMARY

1. All patients who have taken an overdosage of drugs should be admitted to hospital and should have a psychiatric assessment before being discharged.

2. BARBITURATE INTOXICATION

   a. Clinical evidence is more reliable as a guide to the severity of intoxication than the serum barbiturate level.

b. Essentials of management are :—

i. Ensure a clear airway and effective ventilation.

ii. Basic care of the unconscious patient.

iii. Treat hypotension initially by elevating the foot of the bed, but metaraminol or expansion of the blood-volume may occasionally be required.

iv. Force a diuresis if poisoning is severe and there is no contra-indication to this technique.

3. SALICYLATE INTOXICATION

a. Salicylate intoxication may be severe without there being any impairment of consciousness.

b. The serum salicylate level is a reasonably reliable guide to the severity of poisoning.

c. Gastric lavage should always be performed.

d. Forced diuresis is an effective means of aiding salicylate excretion but alkali should not be added to the infusion fluid unless facilities are available for arterial *p*H measurements.

Chapter XIV

GASTRO-INTESTINAL HAEMORRHAGE

SUDDEN haemorrhage from the upper gastro-intestinal tract usually results in haematemesis (the vomiting of blood which may be either fresh or, as the result of digestion, appear similar to coffee grounds) and/or melaena (the passing of tarry black stools per rectum, the appearance of the blood having been altered in transit through the small bowel).

Although the origin of fresh blood passed per rectum may occasionally be a lesion in the upper gastro-intestinal tract, this complaint usually indicates a lesion in the terminal ileum, colon, rectum, or anal canal and will not be discussed further.

Occasionally a patient is seen having fainted following an acute gastro-intestinal bleed but before either a haematemesis or melaena has occurred. A thorough history and physical examination usually clarifies the diagnosis and a rectal examination may be confirmatory by revealing tarry faeces on the finger stall.

All patients who have suffered an acute upper gastro-intestinal haemorrhage should be admitted to hospital, for even if the initial bleed appears trivial it is impossible to predict that a further catastrophic haemorrhage, requiring intensive resuscitation, will not occur in the near future.

It is also advisable to obtain the co-operation of a surgeon in the management of the patient from the time of admission rather than only seeking a surgical opinion when the patient is virtually exsanguinated.

Causes

The common causes of haematemesis and melaena (*Fig.* 8) are:—

1. Chronic duodenal ulcer.

2. Chronic gastric ulcer.

3. Acute gastric erosions. These may be related to the ingestion of aspirin, corticosteroids, or phenylbutazone but often no obvious cause is apparent.

4. Hiatus hernia.

5. Oesophageal varices.

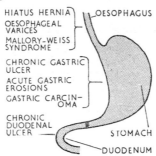

Fig. 8.—Causes of haematemesis and melaena.

Acute gastro-intestinal haemorrhage may occasionally be the presenting feature of carcinoma of the stomach and bleeding may also arise from mucosal tears in the lower oesophagus which result from repeated vomiting regardless of the cause (Mallory-Weiss syndrome).

Other causes which should not be forgotten include the taking of anticoagulant drugs and haemorrhagic disorders such as thrombocytopenia and familial haemorrhagic telangiectasia.

Occasionally, even after full investigation, no cause for the haemorrhage is apparent.

CLINICAL ASPECTS

As previously stated, an acute upper gastro-intestinal haemorrhage usually presents with a haematemesis and/or melaena, often associated with a feeling of faintness or actual loss of consciousness, sweating, palpitations, thirst, and restlessness.

The main problems are to decide:—

1. The cause of the bleeding.
2. The amount of blood lost.

In the drama of the situation it is easy to neglect taking a careful history and making a thorough physical examination, but the emergency is rarely so grave that a few minutes cannot be spared for this purpose and a thorough initial clinical assessment is of considerable importance.

1. CAUSE OF THE BLEEDING

To make an accurate diagnosis of the cause of the bleeding from the history and physical examination alone is only possible in about 50 per cent of cases or less. However, it is often possible to make a shrewd guess and some of the possibilities can at least be excluded with reasonable confidence.

A long history of dyspepsia related to meals suggests a chronic duodenal or gastric ulcer and a detailed analysis of the symptoms may occasionally allow a prediction as

to which is responsible. When a previous barium meal
has been performed the films should be obtained if at all
possible, likewise the details of any prior gastric surgery.

Acute gastric erosions are suggested by an absence of
previous dyspeptic symptoms and a recent history of
alcohol, aspirin, phenylbutazone, or corticosteroid
ingestion. The patient may often forget that he has
recently taken aspirin or he may not regard this as a
drug and fail to mention it when he is asked about this
point. Also he may be unaware that aspirin is a constitu-
ent of a proprietary preparation that he has taken and if
there is any doubt the labelled container should be
obtained and the composition of the preparation
checked.

The possibility of an hiatus hernia is suggested by the
symptom of heartburn occurring on bending down or
lying down at night, occasionally associated with the
regurgitation of gastric contents into the mouth. However, bleeding may also occur from an ulcer in the intra-
thoracic portion of the stomach in a para-oesophageal
hiatus hernia and as the mechanisms which prevent
gastro-oesophageal reflux are not disturbed, heartburn
is not a prominent feature.

Oesophageal varices should be suspected if the spleen is
palpable, for splenomegaly is the most reliable sign of
portal hypertension. Other signs of chronic liver disease
such as jaundice, liver palms, spider naevi, and ascites
may also be apparent. It should be noted, however, that
there is an increased incidence of peptic ulceration in
patients with hepatic cirrhosis so that varices may not
necessarily be the source of the haemorrhage.

Gastric carcinoma is suggested by a recent history of anorexia and weight-loss. Examination occasionally reveals evidence of the gastric lesion itself or hepatomegaly from the presence of metastases.

Careful history-taking and physical examination should exclude the more uncommon causes such as anticoagulant drugs, the Mallory-Weiss syndrome, thrombocytopenia, familial haemorrhagic telangiectasia, etc.

2. ASSESSMENT OF BLOOD-LOSS

This presents some difficulty for the patient's or relative's description of the amount of blood lost is usually unreliable and there is tremendous variation in the response of different patients to the same degree of haemorrhage.

The point at issue is to determine whether or not transfusion is indicated and by comparing the clinical features of haemorrhage with measurement of blood-volume it has been found that this is usually required if:—

  a. The pulse rate is 110/minute or above.

  b. The systolic blood-pressure is 110 mm. Hg or below.

However, a young, fit patient may lose at least 50 per cent of his blood-volume with minimal or no change in the blood-pressure and pulse-rate. In the case of elderly patients, who withstand severe haemorrhage comparatively poorly, it is often wiser to transfuse if significant blood-loss is suspected before a major fall in the blood-pressure occurs.

INVESTIGATIONS

These can be considered under three headings:—

1. CAUSE OF BLEEDING

There is no doubt that the subsequent management of patients with acute gastro-intestinal bleeding is considerably easier if the cause of the haemorrhage is established as early as possible and with this end in view many centres practice endoscopy (oesophagoscopy and/or gastroscopy) and radiology of the upper gastro-intestinal tract (with barium or gastrografin) within a few hours of admission. Such investigations carry no particular hazard in the acute phase and in selected cases can provide extremely valuable information.

The usual practice, however, if the haemorrhage quickly subsides after admission, is to perform a conventional barium swallow and meal examination a few days later and gastroscopy is only performed if there is any definite indication.

If an underlying haemorrhagic disorder is suspected, a platelet count should be performed and the clotting, bleeding, and prothrombin times estimated.

2. ASSESSMENT OF BLOOD-LOSS

Although a base-line haemoglobin and packed cell volume should be obtained, the results are of no value for this purpose since it may take several hours or days for haemodilution to be completed. Nevertheless an initial haemoglobin of 9·0 g./100 ml. or below is a further indication for immediate transfusion.

The technique of measuring the blood-volume using red cells tagged with a radioactive isotope is becoming more widely available and may be of considerable help in this situation. Also measurement of the central venous pressure may be useful in deciding whether systemic arterial hypotension is the result of oligaemia or some other factor.

3. GENERAL INVESTIGATIONS

The blood-urea frequently rises after an acute gastro-intestinal haemorrhage but an excessive elevation (i.e., 100 mg./100 ml. or over), coupled with the presence of protein, casts, or white cells in the urine suggests the presence of coexisting renal disease. A routine electro-cardiogram and chest radiograph are also indicated.

The main value of these investigations is to confirm or exclude any significant coincidental diseases which might have some influence on the decision whether or not surgery should be undertaken if this eventually seems to be indicated.

MANAGEMENT

Many patients stop bleeding soon after admission and no specific measures are required other than a period of careful observation and subsequent investigation in an attempt to establish the cause of the haemorrhage. Bleeding from oesophageal varices is often difficult to control and as gastro-intestinal haemorrhage in chronic liver disease carries the additional risk of precipitating hepatic failure, the management of this problem will be discussed in a separate section at the end of this chapter.

1. CROSS-MATCHING

A blood sample should be taken at the time of admission for haemoglobin estimation and blood grouping and 2 litres of blood should be cross-matched. If this is used, more blood should be cross-matched so that a constant reserve of 1–2 litres is always readily available.

2. OBSERVATION

The pulse and blood-pressure should be recorded half-hourly in addition to noting the general appearance of the patient. The nursing staff should be aware that indications of continuing or recurrent haemorrhage, other than the vomiting of blood or passage of a fresh melaena stool, are:—

a. A falling blood-pressure.

b. Rising pulse-rate.

c. Complaint by the patient of feeling suddenly faint and thirsty associated with signs such as pallor, sweating, and restlessness.

Failure of the nurses to appreciate these points may result in a considerable delay before the house physician is informed that further bleeding has occurred.

3. SEDATION

Patients who have suffered an acute gastro-intestinal haemorrhage are often extremely anxious and some form of sedation is usually required. Morphine is frequently recommended for this purpose but is not the drug of choice. The main use of morphine in clinical medicine is as an analgesic. Severe pain is rarely a feature of gastro-intestinal bleeding and if the patient has complained of recent ulcer pain the release of a large quantity of blood into the stomach usually relieves this symptom. Thus if severe abdominal pain persists after a bleed the possibility of an additional complication, such as perforation, should be suspected and potent analgesics only given when this has been excluded. Other objections to the use of morphine in this situation are:—

a. Morphine has a hypotensive effect and thus reduces the significance of a falling blood-pressure as an indicator of further haemorrhage.

b. Morphine is a potent emetic.

c. Opiates reduce bowel motility and may thus mask the fact that further bleeding has occurred by delaying the appearance of a fresh melaena stool.

Phenobarbitone meets most of these objections and a suitable initial dose is 200 mg. intramuscularly followed by 60 mg. b.d. by mouth.

4. BLOOD TRANSFUSION

As already stated, the widely accepted indications for immediate transfusion are:—

a. Pulse-rate of 110/minute or over.

b. Systolic blood-pressure of 110 mm. Hg or below.

c. An initial haemoglobin of 9·0 g./100 ml. or less.

Blood is transfused until the pulse and blood-pressure return to normal and until the patient looks pink, with warm hands and a full-volume pulse. If there is any doubt as to whether all the blood lost has been replaced, monitoring the central venous pressure can be helpful, as can serial measurements of the blood-volume if the facilities are available.

Occasionally the haemorrhage may be so severe that it is impossible to wait for blood to be cross-matched, even by an abbreviated technique, and under these circumstances there are several alternative methods for urgent restoration of the blood-volume:—

a. The use of unmatched group O Rh negative blood, which is only indicated in cases of extreme urgency.

b. The use of plasma which is an effective substitute for whole blood and is readily available. The great disadvantage of plasma, however, is the possible occurrence of subsequent serum hepatitis. This is often a serious illness and may be fatal.

c. The use of a plasma substitute. Dextran is the most widely used but the infusion of large molecular weight dextran preparations before the withdrawal of blood for cross-matching frequently interferes with compatibility testing. However, macrodex (a dextran preparation with an average molecular weight of 70,000) is free from this complication and is probably the plasma substitute of choice at the present time.

When the rate of blood transfusion is rapid, 10 ml. of 10 per cent calcium gluconate should be given intravenously for every litre of blood transfused. The elevation of the serum potassium by the rapid transfusion of large volumes of stored blood is rarely a problem and can in any case be minimized by the use of as much fresh blood as possible.

helps
(1) overcome citration
(2) helps cardiac function

5. GASTRIC ASPIRATION

This is not usually necessary but if there is any suggestion that the stomach is distended with blood-clot, a naso-oesophageal tube should be passed and the stomach gently lavaged with cold normal saline. The naso-oesophageal tube should then be left in place and aspirated hourly, blood-staining of the aspirate often being the earliest sign that further haemorrhage is occurring.

6. HYDRATION AND NUTRITION

Starvation is contra-indicated and a light diet may safely be given from the time of admission. The maintenance of an adequate state of hydration is also of considerable importance.

7. SURGERY

As stated at the beginning of this chapter, the best management of patients with acute gastro-intestinal haemorrhage is achieved when their supervision is shared jointly between physician and surgeon from the time of admission. The decision as to when surgery should be undertaken for any particular patient is often difficult, although the following are generally accepted indications for operation:—

a. Bleeding from a chronic gastric ulcer.

b. The presence of a duodenal ulcer for many years with either two previous episodes of bleeding, severe symptoms, or evidence of other complications, such as pyloric stenosis.

c. The occurrence of a gastric and duodenal ulcer in the same patient.

d. Any suspicion of a gastric carcinoma.

e. If bleeding is still occurring 48 hours after admission to hospital.

Relative contra-indications are coexisting severe cardiac, respiratory, or renal disease but the factors both for and against surgery must be carefully considered in each individual case.

Emergency Management
of Bleeding Oesophageal Varices

The first essential as described above, is adequate blood transfusion to maintain the circulatory blood-volume.

In addition, the following precautions must be taken to prevent the development of hepatic coma:—

1. The avoidance of morphine as a sedative, phenobarbitone being the drug of choice for this purpose.

2. Oral neomycin (6 g. daily in divided doses) should be given.

3. The colonic contents should be evacuated by enemas.

4. All dietary protein must be stopped and nutrition maintained with glucose to provide 1600 calories per day. This is preferably given orally but may be given via an intragastric tube or as a 20–40 per cent solution infused into the superior or inferior vena cava.

If the bleeding does not stop after adequate transfusion, 20 units of vasopressin in 100 ml. of 5 per cent dextrose solution should be infused intravenously over a period of 10–15 minutes. This method usually enables the haemorrhage to be controlled in approximately 70 per cent of cases but the use of vasopressin carries certain disadvantages:—

a. Vasopressin is a vasoconstrictor and may produce myocardial ischaemia by constriction of the coronary arteries. Thus it is probably best avoided in the elderly and in the presence of known ischaemic heart disease.

b. The effect of vasopressin is frequently only temporary and bleeding often recurs a few hours later. Although the infusion can be repeated, its effectiveness declines each time it is used.

c. The side-effects (colicky abdominal pain and defaecation) are unpleasant but are an inevitable consequence of the infusion of a potent vasopressin preparation.

d. Vasopressin reduces hepatic blood-flow and thus may further impair hepatocellular function.

A less preferable alternative to the use of vasopressin for the control of haemorrhage from oesophageal varices is balloon tamponade using the Sengstaken triple lumen double balloon tube. Before use, the balloons should be checked for any leaks by inflating them underwater. The tube is then lubricated and passed through the mouth into the stomach. The lower balloon is inflated with 200 ml. air and its position in the stomach checked by a plain radiograph of the abdomen. The oesophageal balloon is then distended with air to a pressure of 30 mm. Hg. Traction is exerted on the tube so that the lower balloon compresses the submucous veins in the upper part of the stomach and the oesophageal varices are compressed by the upper balloon. The stomach contents may be aspirated via the third lumen of the tube and repeated pharyngeal suction is also required to remove saliva and other secretions.

Disadvantages of this technique are:—

a. It is extremely distressing for the patient.

b. Upward displacement of the tube may occur with consequent laryngeal obstruction and asphyxia.

c. Ulceration of the lower oesophagus: for this reason the pressure in the balloon should be released after 24–36 hours.

When tamponade is discontinued the bleeding may recur and in this event emergency surgery must be considered. In these circumstances, surgery designed to reduce the portal pressure is hazardous and when liver function is impaired emergency surgery carries a particularly high mortality.

SUMMARY

1. All patients with acute gastro-intestinal bleeding must be admitted to hospital and should preferably be

under the joint supervision of physician and surgeon from the outset.

2. Careful history-taking and physical examination provide valuable information both as to the cause of the bleeding and the amount of blood lost.

3. Blood grouping should be done on all patients and 1–2 litres of blood cross-matched as a routine.

4. Apart from blood transfusion, other important aspects of management are the frequent recording of pulse-rate and blood-pressure, the use of phenobarbitone rather than morphine for sedation, and the consideration of surgery before the patient is exsanguinated.

5. Acute gastro-intestinal haemorrhage in the presence of chronic liver disease carries the additional risk of producing hepatic coma and in this event, oral neomycin should be given in addition to stopping all dietary protein.

6. Intravenous pitressin is preferable to balloon tamponade for the control of bleeding from oesophageal varices but both methods are far from satisfactory. Emergency surgery for this condition is particularly hazardous in the presence of severely impaired liver function.

Chapter XV

DIABETIC KETOSIS

As the result of better education and supervision, severe ketosis now occurs only comparatively infrequently in known diabetics and is more frequently encountered as a presenting feature of patients who were not previously known to suffer from diabetes.

The most common precipitating factor is infection (usually pneumonia, a urinary tract infection, or gastro-enteritis) but diabetic ketosis may also be a consequence of surgery, trauma, or neglect.

The biochemical disturbances stem from the relative lack of insulin which results in inadequate intracellular glucose utilization. Thus hyperglycaemia occurs which, once the renal threshold for glucose has been surpassed, results in an osmotic diuresis with sodium loss as an inevitable concomitant. Increased fatty acid oxidation is also a consequence of inadequate glucose catabolism and results in the formation of excessive amounts of aceto-acetic acid. The usual metabolic pathway for the disposal of this substance becomes grossly overloaded, leading to an accumulation of acid metabolites. Thus a metabolic acidosis results. Hydrogen ions move into the cell in exchange for potassium ions so that a deficit of intracellular potassium occurs.

These disturbances are aggravated by the effects of vomiting and hyperventilation, both frequent features of severe ketoacidosis.

CLINICAL FEATURES

The clinical picture depends on the severity of the ketosis, ranging from the discovery of ketonuria by routine testing in a symptomless patient to an illness of extreme severity.

An important point is that the full clinical picture takes several hours or even days to develop and the onset is never sudden.

Extreme thirst, a dry mouth, and polyuria are usually the initial complaints, followed by anorexia, vomiting, and general prostration. Severe abdominal pain may be prominent. Consciousness is progressively impaired and coma eventually supervenes.

When ketosis and dehydration are severe, physical examination reveals an ill-looking, drowsy, or comatose patient. The respirations are deep and rapid and a strong smell of acetone may be detectable in the breath. The eyes are sunken, the intra-ocular tension reduced, the tongue extremely dry, and the skin loose and inelastic. The pulse is rapid and of poor volume and systemic hypotension eventually occurs.

DIAGNOSIS

Although met with only infrequently, severe diabetic ketosis is rarely confused with any other condition. As stated in the following chapter, the distinction between coma due to ketosis and coma resulting from hypo-glycaemia in a diabetic patient is rarely difficult if the rate of onset of the illness and the general condition of the patient are considered. Salicylate intoxication bears some superficial resemblance to diabetic ketosis but although there may be some reducing substances in the urine in the former condition, significant amounts of glucose are not present. Other metabolic and intracranial causes of coma should be briefly considered but can usually be excluded by thorough physical examination and the basic investigations described below.

INVESTIGATIONS

The diagnosis is confirmed by finding:—

1. Heavy glycosuria and ketonuria (the catheter which is almost invariably necessary to obtain the first urine specimen, should be left in situ so that further urine specimens may be tested for glucose and ketones as frequently as desired).

2. Ketones detectable in the plasma. These may be present in the absence of ketonuria if there is gross dehydration with impaired renal function.

3. Hyperglycaemia—the blood-glucose usually being between 300 and 1000 mg./ml. but higher levels may occasionally be found.

The severity of the condition is assessed by a combination of the clinical features and the following investigations:—

1. The concentration of plasma ketones.

2. Plasma urea and electrolytes. The plasma urea is frequently elevated and the sodium and chloride low but all may be within the normal range. The plasma potassium is usually normal although there may be a considerable

intracellular potassium deficit. The plasma bicarbonate is below 20 mEq./l. and may be less than 10 mEq./l. if ketoacidosis is severe.

3. Haemoglobin and packed cell volume. Both may be elevated if dehydration is severe.

4. Blood pH. This frequently falls to 7·1 and occasionally to below 7·0.

These investigations should be done immediately the patient is admitted to hospital, for apart from confirming the diagnosis and providing an indication as to the severity of the condition, they also serve as a base-line for judging the effectiveness of therapy.

Investigations to discover the precipitating cause are not of great urgency but a chest radiograph and urine examination and culture should be done as soon as possible.

MANAGEMENT

Severe diabetic ketosis is a potentially lethal condition and the prompt commencement of effective therapy is a matter of urgency. The main aims of treatment are:—

1. To control the hyperglycaemia and abolish the ketosis.

2. To correct the dehydration and electrolyte imbalance.

3. To treat the precipitating cause.

A suitable régime is as follows:—

1. INITIAL INSULIN DOSAGE

When the diagnosis has been confirmed by urine testing, an injection of soluble insulin should be given without waiting for the result of the blood investigations. One hundred units is a widely recommended initial dose,

40 units being given intravenously and 60 units by deep intramuscular injection. Large doses of insulin are usually required because ketosis induces a state of insulin resistance. However, if the metabolic acidosis is adequately treated with bicarbonate (*see below*) the insulin requirements are frequently much less and 60–80 units of soluble insulin is a more appropriate initial dose in these circumstances.

2. FLUID REPLACEMENT

An intravenous infusion should be started at the time of admission and normal saline used as the basic infusion fluid. The amount of fluid lost is usually underestimated and anything from 6–8 litres may be required in the first 12 hours. The first litre should be given over 30 minutes and the second over the next hour. The infusion rate can then be slowed to 1 litre every 2–3 hours.

Although this amount of normal saline produces no complications in the majority of patients, there is a risk of producing both sodium and chloride overload in the presence of impaired renal function. If this is suspected therefore, it might be wise to use a solution with a lower sodium and chloride content. Butler's solution (containing 100 mEq. Na^+, 60 mEq. Cl^-, and 40 mEq. HCO_3^- per litre) meets this requirement and has the additional advantage of containing bicarbonate for correction of the acid-base disturbance.

3. ANTICIPATION OF HYPOKALAEMIA

Insulin aids the transfer of potassium into the cells from the extracellular fluid and this often results in a dangerously low serum potassium level a few hours after the commencement of therapy. This fall should be anticipated rather than waiting for its occurrence before giving supplements and, providing renal function is satisfactory, 25 mEq. of potassium should be added to each litre of infusion fluid. Serial serum potassium levels are rarely of much value as a guide to therapy, for gross disturbance of the intracellular potassium may be present and yet the serum level be within the normal range.

4. CORRECTION OF ACID-BASE DISTURBANCE

Metabolic acidosis is indicated clinically by hyperventilation and biochemically by a fall in the plasma bicarbonate and eventually the blood pH. Correction of the acid-base disturbance with bicarbonate leads to quicker recovery and reduces the insulin requirement which would otherwise be needed. When Butler's solution is not being used, 200 mEq. of sodium bicarbonate (i.e., 200 ml. of the Molar solution) can be added to the first litre of normal saline. This may be sufficient but further 100 mEq. aliquots of bicarbonate, again added to the saline infusion, may be given if necessary until there is no clinical evidence of acidosis, the plasma bicarbonate is not less than 20mEq./l., or the blood pH is at least 7·2.

5. GASTRIC ASPIRATION

If the patient is vomiting or deeply comatose a small intragastric tube should be passed and aspirated half-hourly, for gastric and intestinal stasis tends to occur and inhalation of gastric contents is a potential hazard. In consequence, the administration of fluid either orally or via the intragastric tube during severe ketosis is contra-indicated.

6. SUBSEQUENT INSULIN DOSAGE

Further deep intramuscular injections of soluble insulin are given every 2–3 hours, the dose (usually 20–40 units) being regulated by serial blood-glucose estimations until the blood-glucose falls to 300 mg./100 ml. Higher doses are rarely needed when bicarbonate is used to correct the severe acidosis.

When the blood-glucose falls to 300 mg./100 ml. :—

a. Urine testing can replace serial blood-glucose estimations for the regulation of the dose of soluble insulin which should continue to be given at 3–4 hourly intervals. A suitable sliding scale of insulin dosage is :—

Urine Glucose	Dose of Soluble Insulin
2 per cent or above	24 units
1 per cent	16 units
$\frac{3}{4}$ per cent	12 units
$\frac{1}{2}$ per cent	8 units

b. Saline is replaced as the basic infusion fluid by 5 per cent dextrose solution (1 litre 6 hourly, 25 mEq. of potassium being added to each). Hypoglycaemia is likely to occur at this stage and the insulin requirements rapidly diminish. Additional aliquots of 20–50 ml. of 50 per cent glucose may be required if hypoglycaemia develops.

The condition which precipitated the ketosis must be treated if possible. As previously stated, this is usually an infection and appropriate antibiotic therapy is indicated. Even if there is no evidence of infection, penicillin G,

1 mega unit intramuscularly twice daily should be given as a prophylactic measure.

When abdominal pain is a prominent feature it is sometimes difficult to decide if this is a consequence of the ketosis or whether an acute intra-abdominal crisis has precipitated the diabetic emergency. If a detailed history is available it may be apparent that the poor diabetic control preceded the onset of abdominal pain. A white-cell count is of no value in this situation for a leucocytosis occurs in uncomplicated diabetic ketosis and there may still be some doubt after a thorough physical examination and an abdominal ·radiograph. In this event the wisest course is, under antibiotic cover, to treat the ketosis as described and if the pain does not rapidly improve to obtain a surgical opinion.

When the patient's condition has improved to the extent that he is fully conscious and able to take fluids orally, the frequency of the injections of soluble insulin (which can now be given subcutaneously instead of intramuscularly) can be reduced to 4–6 hourly. Glucose, 50 g. orally, is given with each injection, prior to the commencement of thrice daily soluble insulin and normal food.

When the ketosis is less severe, the principles of the treatment are the same but the details are modified to meet the requirements of each individual case, i.e., if the patient is fully conscious and not vomiting, fluid and electrolytes can be given orally, less frequent injections of soluble insulin are required, and the dose can be based on the urine glucose concentration from the beginning if the blood-glucose is 300 mg. or below.

Hyperosmolar Non-ketotic
Diabetic Coma

Coma may occasionally develop in an elderly patient who has previously suffered from mild diabetes, controlled either by dietary restriction alone or with the aid of an oral hypoglycaemic agent. Heavy glycosuria is detected and the blood-glucose grossly elevated, but ketones are absent from the plasma and the plasma bicarbonate is normal or is only minimally reduced. There is invariably evidence of severe dehydration. Hypernatraemia is frequent and this, together with the hyperglycaemia, results in hyperosmolarity of the serum. The essentials of treatment are to lower the blood-glucose, and thus curtail the osmotic diuresis, and to restore fluid balance. The first objective is achieved by the frequent injection of soluble insulin (as described *above*), and the second by the use of large amounts of hypotonic saline solution, for in these circumstances 5 per cent dextrose aggravates the osmotic diuresis and normal saline contains an excessive amount of sodium.

As for severe ketosis, a precipitating cause should be sought and treated where possible. After the emergency is over it is usually again possible to achieve adequate diabetic control without the aid of insulin.

Summary

1. The commonest precipitating factor of diabetic ketosis is infection.

2. The severity of the condition is assessed by a consideration of the clinical features and the results of

the following investigations, which should be made immediately the patient is admitted to hospital:—

a. Blood-glucose.

b. Plasma ketones.

c. Hb. and P.C.V.

d. Plasma urea and electrolytes (including bicarbonate.)

e. Blood *p*H (if possible).

These results also serve as a base-line for judging the effect of therapy.

3. Treatment must be started without delay, the essentials of therapy being:—

a. Insulin—after the first injection subsequent doses are governed by the result of serial blood-glucose estimations until the blood-glucose falls to 300 mg./ 100 ml. At this stage the urinary glucose content can be substituted as a reasonably reliable guide.

b. Adequate fluid replacement.

c. Anticipation of hypokalaemia by the early use of potassium supplements.

d. Correction of the acidosis with bicarbonate.

e. Gastric aspiration if the patient is vomiting or deeply comatose.

4. The precipitating cause must be treated whenever possible. Even if there is no evidence of infection, penicillin should be given prophylactically.

Chapter XVI

HYPOGLYCAEMIA

THE brain, having only an extremely limited ability to store carbohydrate in the form of glycogen, is almost entirely dependent on glucose as its source of energy and is thus very sensitive to hypoglycaemia. This is arbitrarily defined as a blood-glucose level of below 40 mg./ 100 ml., and symptoms of cerebral dysfunction rarely occur until the glucose content of the cerebral arterial blood falls below this level. However, symptoms of hypoglycaemia may occur even though the blood-glucose is normal or only minimally reduced, if there has been a rapid fall from a much higher level.

Severe or recurrent episodes of hypoglycaemia may result in permanent cerebral damage. Thus, treatment of the hypoglycaemic state is urgent and further attacks should be prevented if possible.

CAUSE

Although spontaneous hypoglycaemia may occur, it is comparatively rare and will not be considered here other than to suggest that if a patient is suffering from transient unconscious attacks, the cause of which is obscure, it is well worth taking blood for estimation of the glucose content during such an episode if the opportunity arises.

The problem of hypoglycaemia in clinical practice is mainly confined to diabetic patients receiving insulin therapy, and usually occurs because of one of the following:—

1. The self-administration of a wrong dose of insulin, usually by accident but occasionally by design.

2. A delayed or missed meal.

3. Excessive physical exertion.

MANIFESTATIONS OF HYPOGLYCAEMIA

Early symptoms are sweating, headache, irritability, and inability to concentrate. If the hypoglycaemia is uncorrected, these may be followed by irrational or aggressive behaviour, loss of consciousness, and eventual convulsions.

The physical signs are of two-fold origin:—

1. Those of cerebral dysfunction, i.e., slurred speech and incoordination followed by loss of consciousness, often with bilateral extensor plantar responses. Occasionally other focal neurological signs may be present.

2. Those due to the outpouring of adrenaline from the adrenal medulla, provoked by the low blood-glucose level, i.e., warm, sweaty skin, dilated pupils, and rapid full-volume pulse.

DIAGNOSIS

The diagnosis of an hypoglycaemic episode in a diabetic patient is usually easy and textbook tables, which compare and contrast the manifestations of hypoglycaemia with those of severe diabetic ketosis, suggesting that these two states may often be confused, exaggerate the problem.

If a witness is available who can supply details as to the health and circumstances of the patient prior to his becoming unconscious, the diagnosis is usually obvious. Also, physical examination is extremely helpful, there being a marked difference between an ill-looking, dehydrated, hypotensive patient, smelling strongly of ketones, and one with hypoglycaemia, the signs of which are outlined above.

The diagnosis can easily be confirmed, either by the use of a Dextrostix which gives a quick but only approximate value of the blood-glucose, or by making a conventional blood-glucose estimation. Treatment need not be delayed while the latter is in progress but the result is of great value if the patient fails to recover after therapy and doubts begin to arise about the original diagnosis. In this event, if the basal blood-glucose was low, the treatment has obviously not been effective, but if the initial level was normal alternative diagnoses must be considered.

MANAGEMENT

Glucose is the treatment of choice and usually needs to be given intravenously if the patient is unconscious or too stuporose to swallow. Fifty ml. of a 50 per cent glucose solution are usually required. This has a high viscosity, and valuable minutes will be saved if a wide-bore needle is used to draw it up into the syringe.

The solution, which is extremely irritant in such high concentration, should be injected slowly into a large peripheral vein with care to prevent any leakage into the perivenous tissues. This is usually followed by a quick recovery of the patient but if this does not occur, and the diagnosis is confirmed by a Dextrostix assessment or a basal blood-glucose level estimation, the injection should either be repeated as often as necessary or a continuous intravenous injection of 5 per cent dextrose commenced.

If the patient is seen in the early stages of hypoglycaemia, he may be too aggressive or unco-operative either to take glucose orally or to allow it to be administered intravenously. Glucagon is then very useful, for the patient can usually be restrained for long enough to permit 1·0 mg. to be injected intramuscularly (*Fig.* 9).

Once the patient has recovered he should be given a good meal to prevent a relapse, for glucose is quickly

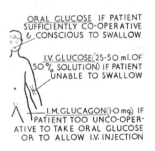

ORAL GLUCOSE IF PATIENT SUFFICIENTLY CO-OPERATIVE & CONSCIOUS TO SWALLOW

I.V. GLUCOSE (25-50 ml. OF 50% SOLUTION) IF PATIENT UNABLE TO SWALLOW

I.M. GLUCAGON (1·0 mg.) IF PATIENT TOO UNCO-OPERATIVE TO TAKE ORAL GLUCOSE OR TO ALLOW I.V. INJECTION

FIG. 9.—Management of hypoglycaemia.

metabolized. Unless the cause of the hypoglycaemic episode is apparent and its repetition preventable (when treatment can be undertaken in the Casualty Department) it is wise, particularly if such attacks are frequent, to admit the patient to hospital in an attempt to achieve more effective diabetic stabilization.

Hypoglycaemia induced by Sulphonylurea Drugs

It is important to realize that severe hypoglycaemia can be induced by the sulphonylureas, and chlorpropamide is most frequently responsible.

Although most of the above remarks apply, diagnosis is often not so easy, for the patient is frequently elderly, the rate of onset much slower, and a cerebrovascular lesion may easily be diagnosed in error, as the frequency of focal neurological signs, which are usually reversible, is much higher.

Treatment is essentially as outlined, but the hypoglycaemia is often prolonged, requiring large amounts of intravenous glucose and frequent injections of glucagon.

In view of this possible complication, elderly patients should be maintained on the lowest possible dose of chlorpropamide necessary to control their diabetes.

Summary

1. Suspect hypoglycaemia in all diabetics on insulin who behave irrationally or are unconscious; also in elderly diabetics on oral hypoglycaemic agents with apparent cerebrovascular lesions.

2. Either a Dextrostix estimation should be performed, or a sample of blood taken for glucose content prior to therapy.

3. Intravenous glucose is the treatment of choice, but glucagon is extremely useful if the patient is uncooperative or the hypoglycaemia sustained.

4. Frequent hypoglycaemic attacks, which carry a risk of producing permanent cerebral damage, necessitate admission to hospital for more effective diabetic stabilization.

GUIDE TO FURTHER READING

THE following sources may be of some use in providing more detailed information concerning the problems discussed in some of the preceding chapters:—

CHAPTER I. MYOCARDIAL INFARCTION
McNICOL, M. W. (1967), 'Intensive Care of the Patient with Acute Myocardial Infarction', *Post-grad. med. J.*, **43,** 207.

CHAPTER III. ACUTE LOWER LIMB ISCHAEMIA
DICKINSON, P. H. (1967), 'The Management of Lower Limb Ischaemia', *Curr. Med. Drugs*, **7,** No. 8, 10.
GILLESPIE, J. A. (1966), 'The Indications for Surgical Treatment of the Ischaemic Leg', *Ibid.*, **7,** No. 1, 3.

CHAPTER IV. DEEP VEIN THROMBOSIS
MARSHALL, R. (1965), *Pulmonary Embolism. Mechanism and Management.* Springfield: Charles C. Thomas.

CHAPTER V. PULMONARY EMBOLISM
BARRITT, D. W. (1964), 'The Diagnosis and Management of Pulmonary Embolism', *Post-grad. med. J.*, **40,** 414.
MARSHALL, R. (1965), *Pulmonary Embolism. Mechanism and Management.* Springfield: Charles C. Thomas.

CHAPTER VI. SPONTANEOUS PNEUMOTHORAX
HORNE, N. W. (1966), 'Spontaneous Pneumothorax: Diagnosis and Management', *Br. med. J.*, **1,** 281.

CHAPTER VII. BRONCHIAL ASTHMA
REES, H. A. (1967), 'Management of Status Asthmaticus', *Post-grad. med. J.*, **43,** 225.
SALTER, R. H. (1967), 'The Management of Severe Bronchial Asthma', *Br. J. clin. Pract.*, **21,** 443.

CHAPTER VIII. ACUTE INFECTIVE EXACERBATION OF CHRONIC BRONCHITIS
CAMPBELL, E. J. M., and HOWELL, J. B. L. (1962), 'Rebreathing Method for Measurement of Mixed Venous P_{CO_2}', *Br. med. J.*, **2,** 630.

McNicol, M. W. (1967), 'The Management of Respiratory Failure', *Hosp. Med.* **1**, 601.

Towers, M. K. (1966), 'Chronic Cor Pulmonale', *Post-grad. med. J.*, **42**, 506.

Chapter IX. Subarachnoid Haemorrhage

Walton, J. N. (1956), *Subarachnoid Haemorrhage*. Edinburgh and London: Livingstone.

Chapter XI. Strokes

Marshall, J. (1965), *The Management of Cerebrovascular Disease*. London: Churchill.

Prineas, J. (1966), 'The Management of Cerebral Infarction', *Curr. Med. Drugs*, **7**, No. 8, 8.

Symposium on Strokes (1967), *Scot. med. J.*, **12** (all the October issue devoted to this problem).

Chapter XII. Transient Unconsciousness

Matthews, W. B. (1963), *Practical Neurology*. Oxford: Blackwell Scientific Publications.

Chapter XIII. Drug Overdosage

Geall, M. (1966), 'The Management of Barbiturate Intoxication', *Hosp. Med.*, **1**, 51.

Graham, J. D. P. (1962), *The Diagnosis and Treatment of Acute Poisoning*. London: Oxford University Press.

Matthew, H., and Lawson, A. A. H. (1966), 'Acute Barbiturate Poisoning—a Review of Two Years Experience', *Q. Jl Med.*, **35**, 539.

Chapter XIV. Gastro-intestinal haemorrhage

Hawkins, C. F. (1963), *Diseases of the Alimentary Tract*. London: Heinemann.

Sherlock, S. (1968), *Diseases of the Liver and Biliary System*, 4th ed. Oxford: Blackwell Scientific Publications.

Chapter XV. Diabetic Ketosis

Pyke, D. A. (ed.) (1962), *Disorders of Carbohydrate Metabolism*. London: Pitman.

Taylor, W. H. (1965), *Fluid Therapy and Disorders of Electrolyte Balance*. Oxford: Blackwell Scientific Publications.

Chapter XVI. Hypoglycaemia

Marks, V., and Rose, F. C. (1965), *Hypoglycaemia*. Oxford: Blackwell Scientific Publications.

INDEX